HEALTH PROMOTION STRATEGIES AND METHODS

SECOND EDITION

NOTICE

Medicine is an ever-changing science. As new research and clinical experience broaden our knowledge, changes in treatment and drug therapy are required. The editors and the publisher of this work have checked with sources believed to be reliable in their efforts to provide information that is complete and generally in accord with the standards accepted at the time of publication. However, in view of the possibility of human error or changes in medical sciences, neither the editors, nor the publisher, nor any other party who has been involved in the preparation or publication of this work warrants that the information contained herein is in every respect accurate or complete. Readers are encouraged to confirm the information contained herein with other sources. For example, and in particular, readers are advised to check the product information sheet included in the package of each drug they plan to administer to be certain that the information contained in this book is accurate and that changes have not been made in the recommended dose or in the contraindications for administration. This recommendation is of particular importance in connection with new or infrequently used drugs.

HEALTH PROMOTION STRATEGIES AND METHODS

SECOND EDITION

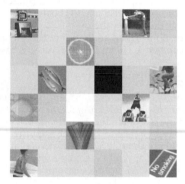

Garry Egger MPH PhD M.A.P.S.

Director, Centre for Health Promotion and Research, Sydney, NSW
Adjunct Professor of Applied Health Promotion, Southern Cross University, Lismore, NSW
Adjunct Professor of Exercise and Nutrition, Deakin University, Melbourne, VIC

Ross Spark MSc PhD

Director, Tropical Public Health Unit Network, Queensland Health, Cairns, QLD

Rob Donovan PhD

Professor of Behavioural Research in Cancer, Curtin University, Perth, WA

The *McGraw-Hill* Companies

Sydney New York San Francisco Auckland
Bangkok Bogotá Caracas Hong Kong
Kuala Lumpur Lisbon London Madrid
Mexico City Milan New Delhi San Juan
Seoul Singapore Taipei Toronto

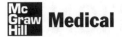
Medical

First edition 1990
Revised 1999
Reprinted 2002
Second edition 2005
Reprinted 2005, 2009

National Library of Australia Cataloguing-in-Publication data:

Egger, Garry.
Health promotion strategies and methods.

2nd ed.
Includes index.
ISBN 9780074715000

1. Health education. 2. Health promotion. I. Spark, Ross. II. Donovan, Rob. III. Title.

613.0994

Published in Australia by
McGraw-Hill Australia Pty Ltd
Level 2, 82 Waterloo Road, North Ryde NSW 2113
Acquisitions Editor: Thu Nguyen
Production Editors: Tess Hardman, Rosemary McDonald
Editor: Cathryn Game
Proofreader: Tim Learner
Indexer: Glenda Browne
Designer (cover and interior): Jan Schmoeger/Designpoint
Cartoonist: Suzanne Plater
Typeset in 9/12 pt Trump Mediaeval by Jan Schmoeger/Designpoint
Printed on 80 gsm woodfree by 1010 Printing International Limited,China

Foreword to the second edition

With its appearance in 1990, the first edition of this book helped to define the field of health promotion strategies and methods. Its balanced approach to individual change, group dynamics, population approaches through mass media and community organisation, and environmental changes through policy initiatives and enforcement earned this book a place in the centre of health promotion. With that balance, it could defend itself in the withering crossfire of the critical, more-rigorous-than-thou scientific reductionism on one side and the rhetoric of the more-equitable-than-thou healthy communities movement on the other.

It could encompass the building-block approach to a health promotion scientifically grounded in theories of health behavioural change and randomised trials that have tested best practices of intervention to change behaviour. At the same time, it offered challenges and experience in broader community interventions and policy changes that could bring about improved conditions of living and environmental supports for people seeking to gain greater control over the determinants of their health. These parameters of the field of health promotion have divided the advocates of opposing ideologically rooted positions and scientifically rigid positions, but their amalgamation in the sweep of this book has made it possible to accommodate both extremes—and the vast middle ground between them.

In the 15 years since the first edition, health promotion has matured scientifically on the behavioural side and has recorded notable successes on the policy and environmental side. The cumulative evidence from patient education and randomised trials of behavioural change has mounted to the point of offering some precision in guidelines for clinical practice of smoking cessation, weight control and other risk factor interventions associated with chronic diseases. At the same time, experience in work sites, schools and communities have been documented with increasing consistency to provide guidance for public health practitioners and policy makers seeking to bring about changes in media and other environments to make them more conducive to health for whole populations.

This second edition reflects these advances in the fledgling science and art of health promotion. It encompasses the spectrum of individual, group, institutional, community and societal strategies and methods for which theory, research and experience have provided a growing base of confidence among health promotion planners and practitioners.

LAWRENCE W. GREEN
Professor, Health Care and Epidemiology, Faculty of Medicine
Director, Institute of Health Promotion Research, Faculty of Graduate Studies
University of British Columbia, Vancouver, BC, Canada

Contents

Acknowledgments

This book is based on materials originally developed for the Distance Education Program of the Postgraduate Diploma in Health Promotion, Curtin University of Technology.

The second edition of *Health Promotion Strategies and Methods* would not have been possible without the help of many individuals and organisations. In particular, the authors would like to thank all those who contributed case studies, ideas and suggestions to this edition. Special thanks go to Suzanne Plater for cartoons and to Dr Gauden Galea and Dr Tommaso Cavalli-Sforza from the World Health Organization's Western Pacific Regional Office for enabling us to put these principles into practice in the Asia-Pacific region.

We are grateful for the support and encouragement provided by a number of organisations, including Queensland Health, VicHealth, the Health Department of Western Australia, the Northern Territory Department of Health and Community Services, the Cancer Council of Western Australia and the School of Public Health at Curtin University of Technology.

We also wish to acknowledge all the individuals and organisations who contributed to the first and revised editions of this book.

About the authors

Professor Garry Egger MPH PhD M.A.P.S. has worked in epidemiology and health promotion in government and industry and as a consultant for the World Health Organisation and governments in Australasia and South-East Asia since 1971. He started the 'GutBusters' men's waist loss program for men in 1991 and 'Professor Trim's Medically Supervised Weight Loss Programs' in 2003. He has conducted academic training in chronic disease management for Australia's general practitioners. Professor Egger wrote the NH&MRC *Guidelines for Physical Activity* and the *Clinical Guidelines for Weight Control and Obesity Management* for doctors. He has written 24 books (including four textbooks) and several scientific articles. In 1978–80 he ran one of the first major health promotion sentinel studies—the Healthy Lifestyle Project—in New South Wales, after which tobacco advertising was restricted in Australia. Dr Egger has appeared on, or written for, most media outlets, including *60 Minutes, Four Corners, A Current Affair, Today Tonight,* the *Sydney Morning Herald,* the *Bulletin* and the *Australian.* He is a council member of the Australian Society for the Study of Obesity (ASSO) and a Fellow of the Australian Council for Health, Physical Education and Recreation (ACHPER).

Dr Ross Spark MSc PhD has been Director of the Tropical Public Health Unit Network for Queensland Health, based in Cairns since 1993. He has spent most of his career in northern Australia, primarily involved in tropical and Indigenous health issues. As senior research fellow in the School of Public Health at Curtin University, Perth (1989–92), he conducted health promotion research in the Kimberley region. Before that he spent five years as Director of Health Promotion Services with the Northern Territory Department of Health in Darwin. He has undergraduate degrees (BEd, BA) from the University of Queensland, an MSc in public health from the University of Oregon and a PhD from the School of Public Health at Curtin University. He holds adjunct academic appointments as associate professor in the School of Public Health at Curtin University, the School of Population Health at the University of Queensland and the School of Public Health and Tropical Medicine at James Cook University. He has also consulted in the Asia–Pacific region in public health and health promotion for AusAID, the Secretariat of Pacific Communities and the World Health Organization.

Professor Rob Donovan PhD (Psychology) is a registered psychologist. He holds the Cancer Council of WA Chair in Behavioural Research and is Director of the Centre for Behavioural Research in Cancer Control in the Division of Health Sciences at Curtin University. He has held marketing positions at the University of Western Australia, Pace University, New York University and the University of Georgia, and has been a visiting scientist at the US Centers for Disease Control and Prevention in Atlanta, Georgia. He has more than 30 years experience in conducting research and developing communication strategies to achieve belief, attitude and behavioural change for Australian governments, NGOs and national brand advertisers. He is author or co-author of more than a hundred journal articles and book chapters in psychology, health and marketing, and has also written or jointly written three books on health promotion, the media and social marketing. In addition to behavioural aspects of cancer control, he has served on the National Expert Advisory Committee on Tobacco (NEACT) and the Australian Health Ministers' National Obesity Taskforce Scientific Reference Group, and is a member of the Western Australian Domestic Violence Campaign Advisory Committee and the World Anti-Doping Agency's Ethics and Education Committee.

Chapter 1
Towards better health

Summary of main points

- There have been big improvements in health in Australia and New Zealand over the last century.
- Lifestyle-related and other chronic diseases continue to increase, and concerns have been raised about the new epidemic of obesity and its associated problems.
- Some infectious diseases that were thought to be a thing of the past have re-emerged, and new infectious diseases are likely to present challenges in future.
- Because of environmental and possible genetic interactions, neighbouring Asian and Pacific countries are even more affected by modern industrialised lifestyles.
- Health promotion is a developing 'art–science' involving processes of individual, social and environmental change as well as health sciences content.
- Health promotion strategies can be aimed at individuals, groups or whole populations. Strategies aimed at whole populations are likely to yield a better return for the health promotion investment.

Changing health patterns

Overall, the health of people throughout the world, as reflected in increased longevity and decreased morbidity, has been improving over time. However, big differences exist both within and between countries according to changing social, economic and environmental factors and the influence of more fixed genetic and cultural factors. In our region, health patterns in developed countries such as Australia and New Zealand need to be considered separately from those of developing nations in the Pacific as these societies are in transition from traditional to developed nations.

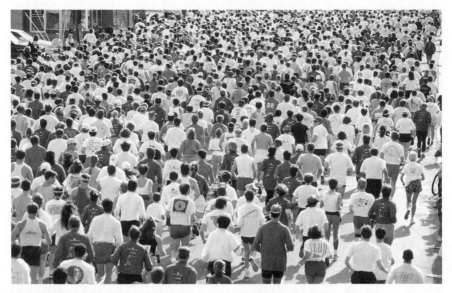

Photo Library

Changing definitions

The change in prominence of different types of disease has led to a confusion of terminology. Initially, a dichotomy was made between communicable and non-communicable diseases (NCDs).[1] The 'diseases of modernity' have typically been labelled non-communicable. However, a recent report (WHO 2004) suggests that 'chronic conditions' is a better overall term. It encompasses certain communicable diseases (i.e. HIV/AIDS, tuberculosis and so on) that, because of advances in treatment methods, have become chronic health problems, along with other chronic diseases such as diabetes, heart disease and cancers, that can't be cured (like acute conditions) but can be managed through organised systems of care to prevent or delay disease complications. In chronic disease management, other allied health professionals, as well as the patient, are as vital as the doctor or nurse for effective health outcomes. Chronic conditions also include long-term mental disorders (such as depression and schizophrenia) and ongoing structural and physical impairments (e.g. blindness, amputations and so on). The terms 'chronic' and 'acute' disease are therefore likely to replace other terms in the future.

Health in Australia and New Zealand

Improvements in health in Australia and New Zealand over the twentieth century occurred in several phases. First, there was a period of increases in life expectancy from 1900 to approximately 1930—largely owing to improvements in the environment and public health, such as better housing, sanitation and education. In a second phase, from the 1930s to the 1970s, there was a levelling of improvements in infectious diseases but a rise in lifestyle-related diseases, which by the mid-1950s had surpassed infectious diseases as the main causes of death. During a third phase, from 1970 to the beginning of the twenty-first century, there has been a recognition of and greater emphasis on these lifestyle diseases along with an increased appreciation of their socio-environmental aetiologies. A fourth phase now appears to be beginning in which old infectious diseases (such as tuberculosis), new strains of influenza and more recent diseases (such as HIV/AIDS, avian flu and SARS—Severe Acute Respiratory Syndrome), as well as new antibiotic-resistant infections, are emerging as a threat to public health (Heymann & Rodier 2004; Plant 1995). Hence there is the potential double jeopardy of rising infectious as well as non-infectious diseases in future. As history has shown, infectious diseases still pose an enormous threat to humanity. The great influenza epidemic of 1918, for example, is thought to have killed between 40 million and 100 million people worldwide. Yet despite vast resources expended on it, an effective treatment for influenza is still unknown.[2] Prevention, early detection and public health measures remain the best (and only) effective forms of management.

Health promotion needs to be cognisant of and responsive to this changing public health landscape. There is little doubt that the highest priorities for health promotion are chronic diseases, such as diabetes, heart disease, injury and preventable cancers, and their respective risk factors (to which, in developed nations like Australia and New Zealand, more than 80 per cent of the burden of disease can be attributed (AIHW 2004a)). However, many of the strategies and methods of health promotion are equally applicable to an integrated public health response for the management and control of communicable and emerging infectious diseases.

Despite some concerns for the future, there have been big improvements in life expectancy over time. In fact, Australians now enjoy one of the highest longevities in the world, being exceeded only by Japan, Iceland and Sweden for men and Japan and France for women (WHO 2004b). At the beginning of the twentieth century, for example, life expectancy was around 55 years for Australian men and 59 years for women. By the 1920s these figures had risen to 59 for men and 63 for women, and by the beginning of the twenty-first century a newborn male could expect to live to 77.4 years on average and a female to 82.6 (AIHW 2004a). The figures for the non-Maori population in New Zealand are similar, although the improvements for the Maori, as for Indigenous Australians, have not been so impressive. Indigenous Australians, for example, can expect to live about twenty years less than their white counterparts, despite some slow improvements in certain areas of Aboriginal health (AIHW 2004b).

A snapshot of Australia's health, 2004

- Cardiovascular disease is still the leading cause of death for both males and females, despite a marked drop in death rates since the late 1960s.
- Cancer ranks second as an overall cause of death, and death rates from cancer fell between 1992 and 2002. However, it now kills more middle-aged Australians than cardiovascular disease.
- Lung cancer caused most cancer deaths (7303) in Australia in 2002, ranking first in males (4760) and a close second to breast cancer in females (2543 lung cancer and 2698 breast cancer).
- Injury death rates have fallen markedly over the past forty years—but injury is still the leading cause of death for people under the age of 45.
- Suicide death rates have gradually decreased in recent years. The rate for 15–24-year-old males in 2002, for example, was the lowest since 1984.
- Around 800 000 Australians are estimated to have a psychiatric condition serious enough to cause disability.
- Diabetes prevalence has more than doubled since the 1980s and is estimated to affect about a million Australian adults.
- Self-reported diabetes among Indigenous Australians in 2001 was almost four times as high as for other Australians.
- Arthritis and other musculoskeletal conditions were estimated to affect more than 6 million Australians (3 in every 10) in 2001.
- Arthritis and other musculoskeletal conditions cause more disability than any other medical condition, affecting about 34 per cent of all people with a disability.
- About 13 000 people were living with HIV/AIDS in Australia in 2002. The number of new cases of AIDS is now relatively stable at 200–250 each year.

AIHW 2004a

The rise in life expectancy in the non-Indigenous population during the twentieth century can largely be attributed to declining perinatal deaths (from 110 deaths per 1000 live births in 1900 to 8.0/1000 in 2002). There has also been a big decline in deaths from infectious diseases. Improvements in individual disease categories are also impressive. For example, since 1970 there has been more than a 50 per cent decline in death rates from cardiovascular disease as well as a decrease in deaths from road traffic crashes and other injuries, respiratory diseases, lung cancer and stroke (AIHW 2004a).

No obvious single factor has caused these changes. Improvements in health care have been postulated as one factor. But equally, improvements in prevention techniques—including changes in certain aspects of lifestyle (altered diet, increased exercise, reductions in smoking, changes in motor-vehicle driver behaviour), combined with environmental interventions and regulatory interventions for better health (e.g. uniform seatbelt legislation, random breath testing, occupational health and safety, and changes in the food supply)—have almost certainly played a part.

Still, despite the gains, there remains considerable opportunity for further improvement and some concern for the future. For example, the incidence of heart disease in Australia, the USA and the UK is still four times that of Japan. Despite early improvements in heart disease death rates owing to smoking declines and improvements in treatment, emerging risk factors, such as obesity and inactivity, have seen a slowing down in improvements in death rates from heart disease. Type 2 diabetes (which is also associated with obesity) is now in epidemic proportions. Because around 80 per cent of diabetic patients will die of heart disease, the rise in diabetes is the main cause of the recent slow-down in improvements in heart disease death rates (Engelgau et al. 2004). Skin cancer, cervical cancer, bowel cancer and lung cancer rates remain high in Australia and New Zealand, and there is still room for improvement in injury rates, such as falls by the elderly and road trauma (AIHW 2004a). There is also continuing concern about the high rates of smoking among adolescents, although recent studies suggest that adolescent smoking rates might have begun to decrease, at least among younger Australian secondary students, while rates among older students might have levelled out (Hill et al. 2002). Finally, there is the worrying rise in severe and new infectious diseases as referred to above.

A review of evidence has shown major changes in public health since the 1960s and 1970s in Australia. Trends observed since the 1990s are shown in table 1.1 on page 6.

Measures of improvement

Another important factor to be considered is the relative emphasis we place on death (mortality) versus illness (morbidity). Historically, medical interventions have focused on treating life-threatening illnesses, which in recent years have been the chronic degenerative diseases, such as stroke, cancer and heart disease. However, we all must die at some time and, in old age, disease that leads to rapid death might be viewed as a good to be sought rather than as an evil to be shunned. It is logical therefore to place more emphasis on preventing the diseases that cause premature death or disability than death *per se*. One way to do so is by using a common metric, the Disability-Adjusted Life Year, or DALY. One DALY is a lost year of healthy life and is calculated as a combination of years of life lost (YLL) owing to premature mortality, and equivalent healthy years of life lost owing to disability (YLD). When these are considered, the picture is somewhat different from simple mortality (see table 1.2). Four of the top fifteen diseases that cause greater DALYs are non-fatal or low-fatality diseases (depression, asthma, osteoarthritis and hearing loss). It is also interesting to note that obesity is not on this list. As obesity

Table 1.1: Changes in health

Improvements	Mixed changes	No or little change	Areas getting worse
Overall mortality (particularly infants)	Poor improvements in lower socioeconomic groups	Premature births	Diabetes
Stroke		Asthma	Obesity and associated metabolic problems (diabetes, fatty liver and so on)
Injury	Chronic Obstructive Pulmonary Disease (COPD)	Illicit drug use	
Road safety		Physical inactivity	
Dental health	Heart disease	Indigenous health	Problems associated with obesity (arthritis, sleep apnoea, respiratory problems and so on)
Congenital abnormalities	Lung cancer	HIV/AIDS	
	Cervical cancer		
Loss of all natural teeth	Skin cancer		Prostate cancer
Vaccine preventable diseases	Breast cancer		Senile dementia
	Youth suicide		Depression
Colorectal cancer			Emerging infectious disease (SARS, Avian flu and so on)
			Health inequalities

is a risk factor for almost all of the diseases listed, it could be regarded as the number 1 contributor to the burden of disease today, and hence needs special consideration in any contemporary analysis of disease trends.

Another, albeit less fully developed, measure of health is 'Quality of Life'. There are several approaches to measuring it, and a single measure has yet to be agreed upon. Although quality of life might be the ultimate measure of good health, this is not yet available (Rogerson 1995).

The rise of obesity

Since the first edition of this text in 1990, obesity has become one of the world's biggest and fastest growing epidemics. More than 67 per cent of Australian men and 55 per cent of women were classified in 2001 as overweight or obese, as measured by a body mass index (BMI)[3] of greater than 25. Around 20 per cent were classified as obese, with a BMI > 30 (International Diabetes Institute 2002). Weight gain in men since the 1990s has averaged around 1.4 g per day and in women around 1.5 g per day (AIHW 2004c). In New Zealand the figures are similar, but in the surrounding countries of the Pacific they are even higher (see page 11).

Table 1.2: The fifteen leading causes of burden of disease (DALYs) and injury in Australia (AIHW 2004a)

Cause of burden of disease	Percentage of total burden
1. Ischaemic heart disease	12.4
2. Stroke	5.4
3. Chronic Obstructive Pulmonary Disease (COPD)	3.7
4. Depression	3.7
5. Lung cancer	3.6
6. Dementia	3.5
7. Diabetes	3.0
8. Colorectal cancer	2.7
9. Asthma	2.6
10. Osteoarthritis	2.2
11. Suicide and self-inflicted injuries	2.2
12. Road traffic accidents	2.2
13. Breast cancer	2.2
14. Hearing loss	1.9
15. Alcohol dependence and harmful use	1.8

Global strategy on diet, physical activity and health

After an initially adverse response from the sugar industry and threats by the US to withdraw funding, the World Health Organization (WHO) released a global strategy on diet, physical activity and health in May 2004.
   The strategy has four main objectives:

1. to reduce the risk factors for non-communicable diseases that stem from unhealthy diets and physical inactivity by means of essential public health action and health-promoting and disease-preventing measures
2. to increase the overall awareness and understanding of the influences of diet and physical activity on health and of the positive impact of preventive interventions
3. to encourage the development, strengthening and implementation of global, regional, national and community policies and action plans

to improve diets and increase physical activity that are sustainable, comprehensive and that actively engage all sectors, including civil society, the private sector and the media

4. to monitor scientific data and key influences on diet and physical activity; to support research in a broad spectrum of relevant areas, including evaluation of interventions; and to strengthen the human resources needed in this domain to enhance and sustain health. Proposals to do this include:

- the role of the WHO in developing strategies, providing guidance, disseminating information and promoting and providing support for training of health professionals
- the need for governments to develop national strategies and guidelines, education, systems for marketing, labelling and promotion of unhealthy products, appropriate food and agriculture policies, programs and partnerships and to provide clear public messages, develop surveillance and research capacity and implement prevention services in schools and the health system.

The full text of the global strategy is available at www.who.int/gb/ebwha/ pdf_files/WHA57/A57_R17-en.pdf

This would not be of concern if obesity was just an aesthetic issue, but research during the 1980s and 1990s has shown a growing list of diseases (at least thirty-five) for which obesity is a leading cause. It is now apparent that obesity is the first visible sign of a range of different problems associated with metabolism, variously known as the 'metabolic syndrome', and with insulin resistance as an underlying cause. More importantly, the epidemic of obesity has spawned a cascade of smaller epidemics, such as diabetes, sleep apnoea, fatty liver, renal failure and joint problems. It is also one of the few diseases that are self-perpetuating because of a number of different vicious cycles. Being overweight can cause joint problems and immobility, which leads an individual to become less active and therefore to gain more weight. Carrying excessive abdominal fatness can lead to metabolic problems, such as insulin resistance, diabetes, gallstones, fatty liver and heart disease. For this reason, waist circumference is now recommended as a standard measure of disease risk (Egger & Binns 2002).

One of the ironies of the obesity epidemic is that it exists even in those developing countries where malnutrition is common, because of the presence of high energy-dense but low nutrient-value processed foods. As obesity is a disease of modernisation, related to the increased availability of energy-dense foods and energy-saving technology, it is unlikely to decrease in the short term, at least in the absence of a major crisis, such as an economic downturn, oil shortage or war. Infectious disease epidemics of the past, such as smallpox, have taken hundreds of years to overcome. This is despite the fact that smallpox and other similar diseases are unpleasant to contract at best and rapidly fatal at worst. The process of contracting obesity on the other hand can be quite pleasant and easy to do (just eat more and move less), and hence it is even less likely to be defeated in the short term. In the meantime, the only significant hope is an increase in individual knowledge—given lower rates of the problem among more highly educated individuals—and changes in obesity-inducing environments.

Determinants of health

There are many factors that influence health in individuals and populations (see figure 1.1). Determinants help to explain and predict trends in health and explain why some groups have better or worse health than others. They are the key to the prevention of disease, illness or injury. Some determinants like cigarette smoking are risk factors whereas others, like healthy food intake, are protective factors. Behavioural factors can be changed, but biological factors, such as age, sex and genetics, generally cannot, although in the case of the latter, much work is being carried out to use genetic knowledge to treat and counsel prospective parents about diseases with a genetic basis.

Determinants have been described as a web of causes with broad causal pathways or 'chains' that affect health (AIHW 2004a), such as those shown in figure 1.1 on page 10.

A small number of risk factors accounts for a significant proportion of diseases, as shown in table 1.3.

Table 1.3: Proportion of total disease burden attributed to 10 selected risk factors based on disability affected life years (DALYs) (AIHW 2004a)

Risk factor	Males (%)	Females (%)
Tobacco smoking	12.1	6.8
Physical inactivity	6.0	7.5
High blood pressure	5.1	5.8
Alcohol harm	6.6	3.1
Alcohol benefit	−2.4	−3.2
Overweight	4.4	4.3
Lack of fruit/veg.	3.0	2.4
High blood cholesterol	3.2	1.9
Illicit drugs	2.2	1.3
Unsafe sex	1.1	0.7

Note: Attributable disability adjusted life years (DALYs) as a proportion of total DALYs. One DALY equals one year of healthy life lost through premature death or living with disability owing to illness or injury.

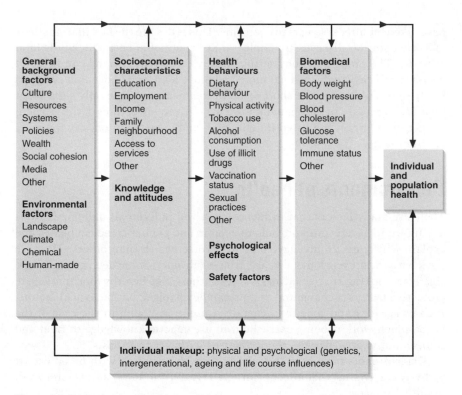

Figure 1.1: Determinants of health
AIHW 2004

The influence of social determinants on health

Although economic development is progressing throughout the world, significant social inequities in health still remain. Socioeconomic status (SES) itself has been shown to be a leading predictor of all causes of disease. Ground-breaking work by Professor Michael Marmot in England and Professor Len Syme in the USA has shown that social differentials are not just confined to differences between the rich and the poor, but form a gradient in all social classes. Marmot and Wilkinson (1999) and Marmot (1999) for example have shown that although the highest grades in employment—the administrative grades—have a mortality about half of the average, professional executives, who are the next grade down, have higher mortality than the administrative grades but lower than clerks, who are the next grade down. The lowest working group has about twice the average mortality. Marmot's work on social determinants has led him to propose 'ten solid facts' relating to social status and health (see box 'The solid facts'). Hence, although opportunistic approaches to health promotion are necessary, it should be recognised that major health shifts could require major social change to reduce health inequalities.

The solid facts

1. People's social and economic circumstances affect health throughout life, so health policy must be linked to the social and economic determinants of health.
2. Stress harms health. Social and psychological circumstances can cause long-term stress.
3. The effects of early development last a lifetime. Ensuring that people have a good start in life involves supporting mothers and young children.
4. Social exclusion creates misery and costs lives.
5. Stress in the workplace increases the risk of disease.
6. Job security increases health, wellbeing and job satisfaction.
7. Friendship, good social relations and strong supportive networks improve health at home, at work and in the community.
8. Individuals turn to alcohol, drugs and tobacco and suffer from their use, but their use is influenced by the wider social setting.
9. Healthy food is a political issue.
10. Healthy transport means reducing driving and encouraging more walking and cycling, backed up by better public transport.

Marmot et al. 1999b

Health in the neighbouring Pacific region

Most countries of the neighbouring Pacific region have developing economics with associated health problems of declining or sporadic infectious diseases, combined with the rising incidence of chronic lifestyle-related diseases of adulthood (WHO 2003b). The cost of dealing with the latter is roughly three times that of dealing with the former (Secretariat of Pacific Communities 2002). Through genetic influences, the populations of the Pacific islands are particularly prone to excessive weight gain and its associated metabolic disorders. Overweight and obesity rates (BMI > 25) range from up to 90 per cent in American Samoa to as low as 12 per cent in men in the Solomon Islands (WHO 2003b). Type 2 diabetes is in epidemic proportions in the region, with Nauru for example having one of the highest recorded rates of obesity and diabetes in the world (Zimmet et al. 2003). There are also rapidly increasing rates of heart disease, hypertension and stroke, along with the associated metabolic problems of kidney disease, circulatory problems, eyesight disorders and certain cancers. Because of declining resources and struggling economies, the immediate health future for this region is bleak, and there is a great need for innovative preventive approaches to halt the escalating costs of treatment, which is set to overtake the gross domestic product of many Pacific island countries.

Case study 1.1

Diabetes management in the King of Tonga

Once categorised by the *Guinness Book of Records* as the heaviest monarch in the world, and with a genetic predisposition to modern diseases, the King of Tonga, King Taufaahau Tupou IV, was diagnosed with type 2 diabetes at the age of 55. At this stage his life expectancy was five to ten years, and he was expected to go through the normal progression from early diagnosis to initial medication to multiple medications—including multiple daily insulin injections—to death. Yet with the assistance of an astute physician, the king was encouraged to lose a massive amount of weight (more than 100 kg) over the next ten years, to become more active through an aerobic and resistance training program, and to change his diet to one with reduced fat intake. At the age of 85, he was still not on diabetic medication and was an inspiration to diabetes sufferers around the world.

The case for prevention

Prevention is often touted as being better than cure, but this belief is not usually supported at government level. Less than 1 per cent of the health budget in Australia at the turn of the millennium was allocated for preventive purposes, despite the fact that up to 30 per cent of diseases are thought to be preventable (Armstrong 1989). Obesity alone is estimated to cost between 5 and 10 per cent of the total health budgets of most Western countries (WHO 1998), yet major government support for obesity control programs is currently lacking. This will have to change as up to 70 per cent of all premature deaths have a possible lifestyle aetiology, and seven of the top ten leading causes of death are lifestyle-related (AIHW 2004a). Taking type 2 diabetes alone, figures show that 7 per cent of the population is now diabetic, and a further 15 per cent is pre-diabetic and has the prospect of progressing to definite diabetes within ten years (International Diabetes Institute 2002). US figures suggest that a diabetic person could cost the health system between $A12000 and $A15000 per year (at 2004 rates) before death (Brown et al. 2001), and that of children born in 2000, one in three can be expected to become diabetic within their lifetime (Engelgau et al. 2004). Yet up to 95 per cent of type 2 diabetes is preventable (Hu et al. 2001). Resources therefore will have to be diverted to, or increased at, the front end of diabetes treatment (i.e. prevention) if future health systems (and economies) are to survive.

It has been estimated that of the 30 per cent decline in all causes of mortality since the 1960s, around half can be attributable to prevention of some kind (Egger 1990). In year 2000 dollars this represents a direct and indirect cost saving of around $5 billion per annum, or around 8 per cent of the annual health budget. Reasons for the successes in reductions of smoking, road injury, cardiovascular disease, and control of AIDS/HIV and asthma have all been

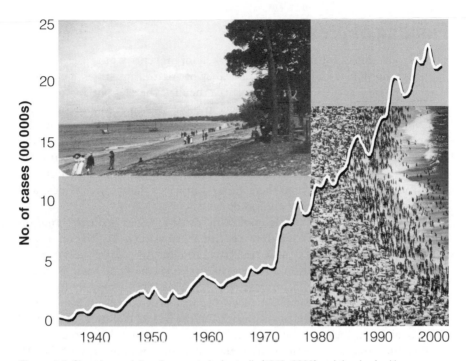

Figure 1.2: Changing social environments in Australia (1940–2000) and the rise in skin cancer
Pictures courtesy of Professor Adele Green, Queensland Institute of Medical Research

detailed in a 1996 report of the National Health and Medical Research Council (NH&MRC 1996).

Prevention also needs to be seen in the context of modern disease progression. 'Primary prevention' refers to initiatives aimed at healthy people before any risk factors emerge and is designed to prevent any progression to disease. 'Secondary prevention' is focused on disease risk factors and early stage disease with the intention of stopping further progression or with returning the individual to a healthy status. 'Tertiary prevention' refers to actions to prevent progression to complications of disease and reoccurrence, and it can include rehabilitation. The focus in this text is on primary and secondary prevention.

Avoidable deaths and phases of prevention

A recent analysis of trends in avoidable deaths in New South Wales from 1980 to 2000 has shown that about half of the potentially avoidable deaths are preventable through primary prevention, a quarter through secondary prevention (mainly heart disease, stroke and colorectal cancer) and a quarter through tertiary prevention and rehabilitation (mainly ischaemic heart disease).

NSW Health 2002

Funding of prevention

The introduction of tobacco taxes earmarked for preventive purposes through health promotion foundations in a number of Australian states has meant a massive increase in funds for preventive health, thereby putting pressure on prevention specialists to provide accountable strategies and methods for carrying out preventive health activities (Carroll 2003). Prevention is generally cheaper than treatment, although its benefits might not always accrue in the short term, and its effects are not always immediately obvious or politically expedient. There are more political votes in the bricks and mortar of hospitals and illness-care facilities than there are in initiatives that prevent illness and premature death—and hence are less obvious.

The increased use of visible marketing techniques in health promotion during the 1980s and 1990s has drawn political attention to health promotion. Preventive campaigns (e.g. quit smoking, condom use, drink-driving and physical activity promotion advertisements) have become visible in the media, and are therefore of interest to politicians. Unfortunately, this has had positive and negative consequences. Because preventive actions are now more visible, more money is forthcoming. But the lack of technical knowledge about health promotion at the political level has sometimes led to the misuse of those resources, for example by equating health promotion with health advertising and engaging advertising agencies without specialised skills in health promotion.

What is health promotion?

In the past, prevention has encompassed changes in public health, including simple environmental interventions, such as John Snow's removal of the handle of the Broad Street pump in the London cholera epidemic of 1849. As people began to congregate in towns and cities, health education arose from a need to transmit information to the public about hygiene and other health-related issues. Now, because many modern diseases have a social, economic, behavioural, environmental or lifestyle aetiology, the emphasis in prevention has shifted to procedures aimed at altering social and physical environments and individual and community behaviour, a process now called health promotion.

Until recently, health promotion was more commonly known by the term 'health education'. Health education emphasised the structuring of learning experiences to facilitate voluntary actions conducive to health (Green et al. 1980). Some writers consider the two terms to be synonymous (Steckler et al. 1995), but we distinguish between the two. Health education is embedded within the broader field of health promotion. Health promotion has been defined as 'the combination of educational and environmental supports for actions and conditions of living conducive to health' (Green & Kreuter 1991).

The changing nature of health promotion

Because behaviour was implicated initially as the immediate cause of many of the modern lifestyle-related diseases, the initial response to dealing with it typically came from established psychological theory, which, by its nature, is individually oriented. However, early writings from the 1970s (e.g. McKeown 1976) and beyond changed the emphasis to a wider scale, which required sociopolitical attributions and the involvement of a number of different disciplines. The Lalonde Report in 1980, for example (Green et al. 1980), introduced into public policy the notion that all causes of death and disease have four contributing elements:

- inadequacies of the existing health-care system
- behavioural factors and unhealthy lifestyles
- environmental hazards, and
- human biological factors.

The central message of the Lalonde Report was that improvements in environments and in the lifestyles of individuals would be the single most effective means of reducing mortality and morbidity.

The 1970s also saw a paradigm shift in thinking in relation to prevention when an American engineer, Dr William Haddon, applied a traditional epidemiological approach to what was considered an intractable problem: injury (Haddon 1980). Haddon recognised the importance of the host, vector and environment, which had for years made up the three corners of an epidemiological triad that was used as the basis for dealing with infectious disease epidemics (figure 1.3). He then applied this to motor vehicle injuries by covering all aspects: education of drivers (hosts), engineering of roads (environments) and modification of vectors (speed). This was also done over time, such that pre-event, event and post-event stages were drawn up in a matrix illustrating options for intervention at all stages. Since then other behavioural epidemics, such as smoking and heart disease, have been aided by this approach. There are current moves to apply this approach to obesity (Egger, Swinburn & Rossner 2003). Figure 1.3 on page 16 shows the epidemiological triad and classical means of dealing with each corner of it.

The 1980s saw health promotion given a higher profile and a more comprehensive and intersectoral role within a 'new public health'. This involved a broader definition of health promotion that encompassed primary health care, public health activities within the health sector and public policy in health and other sectors. The WHO-sponsored Ottawa Charter in 1986 was a milestone in international recognition of health promotion. It outlined five specific actions for health promotion under the new public health. These were:

- developing healthy public policy
- developing personal skills

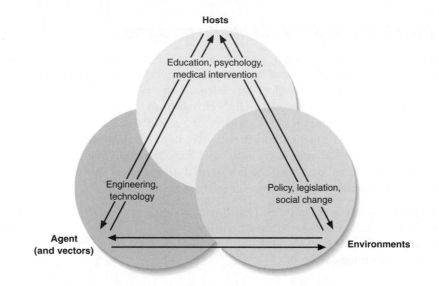

Figure 1.3: The epidemiological triad and approaches to dealing with each corner

- strengthening community action
- creating supportive environments, and
- reorienting health services.

Since then, the Jakarta Declaration (WHO 1997) has added to and refined these original proposals with the following priorities:

- promoting social responsibility for health
- increasing investments for health developments in all sectors
- consolidating and expanding partnerships for health
- increasing community capacity and empowering the individual, and
- securing an infrastructure for health promotion.

A framework for health promotion

As a relatively new field, health promotion has yet to achieve a universally agreed framework of operation for achieving the goals specified above. Indeed, this might not be possible given the dynamic nature of the profession. However, a range of approaches is currently used (including the epidemiological triad described above), varying in focus from dealing with specific health issues (e.g. smoking, drug use, inactivity, weight loss) to focusing on settings (e.g. schools, workplaces, villages) and sectors (e.g. industries, government agencies), or even broader social change (e.g. political and economic action to reduce health inequalities).

Figure 1.4 presents a framework on which the structure of this text is based. We have chosen to focus on individuals, groups or populations to demonstrate the strategies and tools of health promotion practitioners. The strategies range from educational and motivational approaches and social marketing techniques to economic, regulatory, technological and organisational interventions. The first two of these primarily address intra- and interpersonal factors that underlie risks for health, whereas the last four are aimed at the sociopolitical, physical or sociocultural environments—addressing the risk conditions for health. Although these strategies can be used singly, research indicates that health promotion interventions are more likely to be effective where combinations of strategies are employed (Steckler et al. 1995).

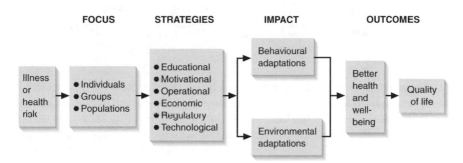

Figure 1.4: A framework for health promotion

The role of the health promotion practitioner

Health promotion, as an emerging discipline, has been clouded by competing philosophies and theories, by battles for professional territory and by fights for government funds. Different players in this game have been adversely labelled as following a medical model or, equally adversely, as following an unscientific social or a political model. This has sometimes led to a dilemma of professional identity for those working in the field.

In the past, health promotion practitioners have been drawn from a variety of different backgrounds: social and behavioural sciences, medicine, politics, nursing, social welfare and community development. Indeed, many of these disciplines regard health promotion as a small but significant part of their service. The advent of specialist tertiary training in health promotion is beginning to define more clearly the role of the full-time health promotion practitioner. Yet the diversity of professional backgrounds from which people come to health promotion remains one of the strengths of this field.

The modern health promotion practitioner is now most likely to be part of an interdisciplinary team with the common goals of increasing total health and wellbeing and decreasing illness in individuals and the broader community. It is not enough for health promotion practitioners to be knowledgeable about matters that influence the individual's health. Their responsibilities also are to modify the health environment.

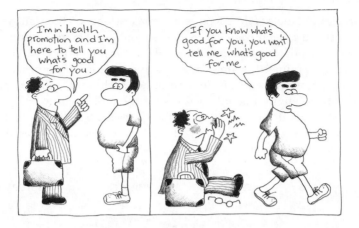

To achieve these aims, the professional health promotion practitioner needs to be skilled in both process and content. Historically, the emphasis has been on the body of health information to be communicated; that is, on content. Equally important are the means of influencing desired change; that is, process. For example, to improve a community's health through changes in nutrition requires an ability to use processes to influence dietary behaviour in line with the content of scientific information available on the benefits of such a change and in the context of broader sociocultural influences (see the box 'Changes in Australian society relevant to the development of health promotion strategy').

Changes in Australian society relevant to the development of health promotion strategy

Changes in Australian society since the 1980s—identified from published statistics (mainly by the Australian Bureau of Statistics) indicate seven area of changes (list below) as being relevant to the development of health promotion strategy.

1. Gender roles and age changes

Women are now leading a dual life as professionals and mothers. From 1992 to 2002 the percentage of families with children younger than 15 in which both parents are employed has risen from 51.8 per cent to 57.1 per cent. Women are also having children later: almost 18 per cent of births were to mothers older than 35 in 2002 compared with less than 11 per cent in 1992. The population is also ageing: the median age increased by almost three years to 35.4 from 1991 to 2001.

2. Changes in household composition

Between 1986 and 2001, the number of one-parent families in Australia increased by 53 per cent. The median age at first marriage had increased by approximately two years to 28.7 in men and 26.9 in women, and there was a rise from 51.7 per cent to 57.1 per cent of two-parent families with children younger than 15 who now work. There was also a 64 per cent increase in the number of people who live alone. Fewer people are getting married, and more childbirths are occurring outside marriage.

3. The influence of immigration

Those born overseas make up 23 per cent of the Australian population, but this proportion hasn't changed since the 1990s. With declining birthrates, the net effect of overseas migration to total growth has increased by almost two-thirds to 53.6 per cent in the decade from 1991 to 2001. The source of origin of immigrants is slowly changing, however, with an increasing number—although still only a small percentage (5.5 per cent)—coming from Asia.

4. Increasing urbanisation

Despite having some of the remotest areas in the world, Australia appears to be becoming more and more urbanised: the population in inner regional areas increased by 14 per cent from 1991 to 2001. More than two-thirds of the population now live in major cities, and 31 per cent live in inner and outer regional areas. Eighty-three per cent of those born overseas live in major cities, but only 31 per cent of the Indigenous population live in cities, 49 per cent living in outer regional, remote and very remote parts of the country.

5. Changes in shopping patterns

Small local shopping units have given way to larger depersonalised centres.

6. Use of computers and the Internet

Perhaps the biggest social trend to occur in modern times is the growth in the use of computers, and particularly the Internet. In 2001, 44 per cent of people had used a home computer and 29 per cent had accessed the Internet from home. A decade before, the Internet was relatively unknown. The use of these time-saving and time-using forms of technology has undoubtedly contributed to the big rapid decline in daily energy expenditure of Australians, which is now estimated to be around two-thirds less than that of a century ago (Vogels et al. 2004).

---

7. Increased environmental and health consciousness

Up to 15 per cent of the population now considers health as an issue in buying food, compared with 5 per cent in the early 1980s. Environmental concerns have also increased dramatically in the same period.

Australian Bureau of Statistics 2003

Unlike the science of medicine, in which a drug discovery can have a continuing influence on health for many years, and where clinical areas are becoming more and more specialised, health promotion needs to monitor and respond to the dynamically changing needs, attitudes, fears and mores of a society. Because health promotion programs take time to plan and put into action, the health promotion practitioner not only must be aware of the community's current trends, but also must possess an ability to chart the direction in which community trends are likely to move in future. To this extent health promotion is both art and science. Determining health risk is a science. Communicating that risk information is an art.

Strategies and methods in health promotion

A strategy in health promotion as described in the rest of this text is 'a plan of action that anticipates barriers and resources in relation to achieving a specific objective' (Green & Kreuter 1991). A method is a tactic employed as part of a strategy. Methods describe the means by which change is to be brought about within the target group. Although some writers use the terms 'methods' and 'strategies' interchangeably, there are distinctions that are relevant to the understanding of the development of health promotion programs.

Strategies

Strategies can be broadly based—such as introducing regulatory changes conducive to healthy behaviour—or relatively narrowly focused—such as changing workplace smoking policy. Within these strategies, there might be a number of methods of achieving the goals of improved health.

Currently, two major strategy dichotomies have influenced the practice of health promotion. The first concerns the emphasis on socioenvironmental change versus individual change. The second concerns the emphasis on high-risk individuals versus whole populations, where risk is averaged out.

Socioenvironmental versus individual behavioural strategies

The socioenvironmental versus individual behaviourist debate concerns notions of the role of individuals in determining their health in contrast to the effect of broader environmental influences.

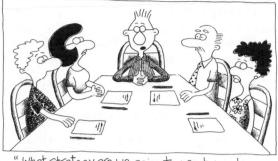

" What strategy are we going to use to work
out what strategy we're going to use?"

The *socioenvironmental interpretation* places the blame for illness among disadvantaged groups on their comparative social and economic deprivation. Strategies for dealing with this are seen as addressing the causes of this deprivation, including poverty, lack of education, unemployment and social factors. This involves 'targeting the system' rather than 'blaming the victim'.

The *individualist interpretation* places emphasis on the responsibility of individuals for their health status. According to this view, health-compromising behaviour by individuals is the main factor causing ill-health. This is based on epidemiological studies, which show that most premature deaths from the major non-communicable diseases (such as coronary heart disease, cancer and stroke) can be attributed to lifestyle factors, known as risk factors. These include smoking, high-fat diets, hypertension, inactivity and stress. This approach suggests that individuals adopt health-compromising behaviour because they have inadequate information, a lack of skills or a negative attitude. The strategies called for here are programs aimed at changing individual behaviour, without specific emphasis on structural factors that could be seen as underlying the causes of behaviour.

In reality, both approaches should be incorporated into programs, as in the more recent syntheses of strategies based on a population perspective (Sallis & Owen 1996; Egger & Swinburn 1996). This synthesis approach focuses attention on both individual and socioenvironmental factors as targets for health promotion interventions. It addresses the importance of interventions directed at changing interpersonal, organisational, community and public policy factors that support and maintain healthy behaviour. The approach assumes that appropriate changes in the social environment will produce changes in individuals, and that the support of individuals in the population is essential for implementing environmental changes.

High risk versus low risk (or whole population strategies)

The high risk versus low risk debate was sparked by English epidemiologist Dr Geoffrey Rose (1992), who asked the question: should we be dealing with sick individuals or sick populations? In essence, the question implies that 'a large number of people at a small risk may give rise to more cases of disease than a small number who are at high risk'. This is also known as the 'prevention paradox'. The corresponding strategies are:

- the *high risk* approach, which seeks to protect susceptible individuals, and
- the *population* approach, which seeks to control the causes of incidence.

According to Rose (1992), 'the two approaches are not usually in competition, but the prior concern should always be to discover and control the causes of incidence'.

A combined high and low risk approach is, in most circumstances and with respect to most health issues, the preferred option. The main principles and strategies for health promotion in this respect include the following components:

- altering the characteristics of lifestyle and environment that are the underlying causes of mass disease (prevention in whole populations)
- preventing the development in low-incidence countries of these precursors (primary prevention in whole populations), and
- within a population, identifying and helping individuals at special risk (high-risk strategy), as well as preventing progression of disease (secondary prevention).

The strategies covered in this book will consider individuals, groups and whole populations. Within these three areas a wide range of methods is available for the implementation of health promotion programs. It should be stressed that effective health promotion requires this variety of methods; for example the more complex the concept, the wider the range of methods that could be needed to apply the concept. In essence, the health promotion practitioner needs to be a 'specialist in generalisation' with some knowledge of the content (and knowledge of where to find greater content expertise and information), as well as knowledge of a wide variety of the processes involved in delivering such content.

Methods

Methods are tactics by which change is brought about within a target group. For example community development and mass media are two methods used to describe a host of activities aimed at modifying health behaviour within the realm of community strategies.

Activities are the specific applications of the methods selected. For example, whereas electronic media could be a method used to effect a change in community behaviour, the production of a poster, a video or a television commercial would be activities using this method.

Some health promotion practitioners choose to specialise in certain methods. Indeed, there is a case for encouraging specialisation in certain methods in order to capitalise on and develop specialist talents. However, it should be acknowledged that this does not imply that any one method is inherently superior or can be applied equally to all health promotion situations.

Career opportunities in health promotion

Opportunities in health promotion have expanded in recent years as a result of the greater emphasis on preventable causes of disease. This has meant not only the advent of health promotion as a profession but also the inclusion of health promotion skills in the roles of other health professionals, such as doctors, nurses, occupational therapists, dentists, teachers, dietitians, exercise specialists, psychologists and many more. Changes in roles mean that employment possibilities can range from clinical practice in the various professions to work in state and federal departments of health and sport and recreation or local government, or to work in segments of the private sector, such as health insurance, hospitals, advertising, food or fitness. At the international level, the World Health Organization, South Pacific Commission, AUSAID, welfare and other aid groups all require personnel with health promotion expertise.

Notes

1 The terms *communicable* and *infectious* have often been used interchangeably, although strictly speaking this is not correct. Some infectious diseases (such as tetanus) might not be communicable (i.e. transmissible from person to person via such things as a food or vector). Communicable diseases, on the other hand, are by definition always infectious and transmissible.
2 For a detailed chronology of the influenza epidemic of 1918 and the lessons to be learned from this for health promotion, see Barry JM, *The Great Influenza*, NY, Viking, 2004.
3 Body Mass Index is measured by weight (in kg) divided by height (in metres)^2.

References

AIHW (Australian Institute of Health and Welfare), 2004a , *The Burden of Disease and Injury in Australia*, AIHW, Canberra.
—— 2004b, *Australia's Health 2004: The Ninth Biennial Report of the Australian Institute of Health and Welfare*, Cat. No. Aus 44, AIHW, Canberra.

—— 2004c, *Health, Wellbeing and Body Weight*, AIHW Bulletin, Issue 13, March.

Armstrong, B. K., 1989, 'Morbidity and mortality in Australia—how much is preventable?', paper presented to the Western Australian Professional Health Educators' Association, Perth, WA.

Australian Bureau of Statistics, 2003, *Australian Social Trends*, ABS, Canberra.

Brown, J. B, Nichols, G. A., Glauber, H. S., Bakst, A. W., Schaeffer, M., & Kelleher, C. C., 2001, 'Health care costs associated with escalation of drug treatment in type 2 diabetes mellitus', *Am J Health-Syst Pharm* 58(2):151–7.

Carroll, A., 2003, *Taxing Sin for Health: A Report Commissioned by the Western Pacific Regional Office of the World Health Organization*, WHO Report, Geneva.

Egger, G., 1990, 'The contribution of prevention to the changing health status of Australians since 1960'. A discussion paper prepared for the Better Health Program, NSW Health Department, Sydney.

Egger, G., & Binns, A., 2002, *The Expert's Weight Loss Guide*, Allen & Unwin, Sydney.

Egger, G., & Swinburn, B., 1996, 'An ecological model for understanding the obesity pandemic', *Brit Med J* 20:227–31.

Egger, G., Swinburn, B., & Rossner, S., 2003, 'Dusting off the epidemiological triad: could it apply to obesity?', *Obes Rev* 4(2):115–20.

Engelgau, M. M., Geiss, L. S., Saaddine, J. B., Boyle, J. P., Benjamin, S. M., Gregg, E. W., Tierney, E. F., Rios-Burrows, N., Mokdad, A. H., Ford, E. S., Imperatore, G., & Venkat Narayan, K. M., 2004, 'The evolving diabetes burden in the United States', *Ann Int Med* 140(11):945–50.

Green, L. W., & Kreuter, M. W., 1991, *Health Promotion Planning: An Educational and Environmental Approach*, Mayfield Publishing Co., Mountain View, Calif.

Green, L. W., Kreuter, M. W., Deeds, S. G., & Partridge, K. B., 1980, *Health Education Planning: A Diagnostic Approach*, Mayfield Publishing Co., Palo Alto, Calif.

Haddon, W., 1980, 'Advances in the epidemiology of injuries as a basis for public policy', *Pub Health Rep* 95:411–21.

Heymann, D. L., & Rodier, G., 2004, 'Global surveillance, national surveillance, and SARS', *Emerg Infect Dis* 10(2):173–5.

Hill, D., White, V., & Effendi, Y., 2002, 'Changes in the use of tobacco among Australian secondary students: results of the 1999 prevalence study and comparisons with earlier years', *Aust NZ J Public Health* 26:156–63.

Hu, F. B., Manson, J. E., Stampfer, M. J., Colditz, G., Liu, S., Solomon, C. G., & Willett, W. C., 2001, 'Diet, lifestyle, and the risk of type 2 diabetes mellitus in women', *N Engl J Med* 345(11):790–7.

International Diabetes Institute, 2002, *Diabetes in Australia*, IDI and NH&MRC Report, Melbourne.

Marmot, M., 1999, 'The solid facts: the social determinants of health', *Health Prom J Aust* 9(2):133–9.

Marmot, M., & Wilkinson, R. G., 1999, *Social Determinants of Health*, Oxford University Press, Oxford.

McKeown, T., 1976, *The Role of Medicine: Dream, Mirage or Nemesis*, Nuffield Provincial Hospitals Trust, London.

NH&MRC (National Health and Medical Research Council), 1996, *Promoting the Health of Australians: Case Studies of Achievements in Improving the Health of the Population*, AGPS, Canberra.

NSW Health (Public Health Division), 2002, *The Health of the People of NSW: A Report of the Chief Health Officer*, NSW Health, Sydney.

Plant, A., 1995, 'Emerging infectious diseases: what should Australia do?', *Aust J Pub Health* 19(6):541–2.

Rogerson, R. J., 1995, 'Environmental and health-related quality of life: conceptual and methodological similarities', *Soc Sci Med* 41(1):1373–82.

Rose, G., 1992, *The Strategy of Preventive Medicine*, Oxford University Press, Oxford.

Sallis, J., & Owen, N., 1996, 'Ecological models', in Glantz, K., Lewis, F. M., & Rimer, B. K. (eds), *Health Behaviour and Health Education: Theory and Practice* (2nd edn), Josscy-Bass, San Francisco, pp. 403–24.

Secretariat of Pacific Communication, 2002, *Obesity in the Pacific: Too Big to Ignore*, SPC Publications, Noumea.

Steckler, A., Allegrante, J. P., Altman, D., Brown, R., Burdine, J. N., Goodman, R. M., & Jorgensen, C. J., 1995, 'Health education intervention strategies: recommendations for future research', *Health Ed Quart* 22(3):307–28.

Vogels, N., Plasqui, G., Egger, G., & Westerterp, K., 2004, 'Secular trends in physical activity: implications for health interventions', *Int J Sports Med* Nov 2004.

WHO (World Health Organization), 1997, *New Players for a New Era: Leading Health Promotion into the 21st Century*, Jakarta Declaration, WHO, Geneva.

—— 1998, *Obesity: Preventing and Managing the Global Epidemic*. Report of WHO Consultation on Obesity, WHO Publications, Geneva.

—— 2003a, *Ministerial Round Table on Diet, Physical Activity and Health*. Regional Committee for the Western Pacific, 53rd Session, Kyoto, Japan, 2002. WHO Publication (WT 500), Geneva.

—— 2003b, *Diet, Food Supply and Obesity in the Pacific*, WHO Publications (WA 695), Geneva.

—— 2004, *The World Health Report 2003*, WHO, Geneva, www.who.int/whr/2003/en/Annex4-en.pdf (viewed 1 March 2004).

Zimmet, P., Shaw, J., & Alberti, K. G., 2003, 'Preventing type 2 diabetes and the dysmetabolic syndrome in the real world: a realistic view', *Diab Med* 20(9):693–702.

Chapter 2
Health and human behaviour

Summary of main points

- Knowledge of risks alone is generally not sufficient to motivate cessation of unhealthy behaviour and adoption of healthy alternatives.
- Various models of attitude and behaviour change have been proposed to explain and describe people's decision making.
- These models are generally based on people's beliefs about the consequences of behaving in certain ways, beliefs about others' endorsement or otherwise of such behaviour, their evaluation of the consequences and relevant others; beliefs about the costs and benefits of alternative behaviour, and beliefs about their capabilities in adopting the healthy alternatives.
- The models provide frameworks for formative research, communication strategies and broader interventions.
- The strategies following from these models can be applied to individuals in one-on-one situations, to groups of varying sizes and to larger populations through mass media and other channels.

The practical value of theory

It's been said that there's nothing more practical than a good theory. Since one goal of health promotion is to change behaviour, an understanding of the behaviour change process is essential if health promotion strategies are to succeed.

Human behaviour, and especially health behaviour, is complex and not always readily understandable. Many theories have been devised in an attempt to explain behaviour. Some are relevant to the study of health, some are not (see Nutbeam & Harris 2004). There is still no unifying theory that comfortably encompasses all those aspects of human behaviour that go to explain health. Indeed, many theories are contradictory and lead to different conclusions under different circumstances. Methods of facilitating behaviour change have also had mixed results.

Because part of the role of the health promotion practitioner is to motivate people towards patterns that will enhance their health, it is important that these theoretical frameworks, however imperfect, are understood and utilised in the selection of strategies and methods. In particular, the practitioner should have a working knowledge of factors that motivate behaviour.

What motivates health behaviour?

Intentions to adopt healthy behaviour, like any other type of behaviour, are motivated or 'triggered' by stimuli in an individual's environment. However, individual responses to such stimuli might or might not relate to health enhancement. For example, the inability to climb a set of stairs without puffing might encourage one individual to seek a higher level of fitness, but encourage another to look for the lifts.

Similarly, health-enhancing behaviour might be adopted for motivations other than to improve health. For example, it is generally believed that more than 60 per cent of those who start an exercise program do so for aesthetic reasons—to lose weight, look good or shape up. Interestingly, those who continue to exercise (only about a third of those who start will continue for longer than three months) tend do so for psychological rather than physical reasons; that is, because it feels good mentally (Donovan & Francas 1990; Lee & Owen 1986).

This opens a second dimension to motivation for health behaviour: the fact that it is dynamic, not static, and might reflect the stage an individual has achieved in adopting and developing a type of behaviour.

The concept of individual risk

In theories of individual behaviour, the level of risk of injury or disease involved is a key factor thought to influence the individual's response when faced with a decision concerning behaviour that might lead to ill-health. Harper, Holman and Dawes (1994) define risk in terms of health in the following way:

> The concept of risk is based on the existence of an association between disease and some attribute or risk factor. In a group of people who all share the same risk factor, the incidence of disease is greater than would occur in the absence of the risk factor. Although a larger proportion of the group than expected develop the disease, there are many who remain disease free. A common example of this is the occurrence of lung cancer among smokers. Along with cases of lung cancer are many smokers who never develop the disease. There are also people who have never smoked, but who nevertheless develop lung cancer, albeit less often than in smokers.
>
> Risk implies only association and not causation. This is not to say that some risk factors—for example, irradiation, asbestos, or cigarettes—are not causative agents. A risk factor, in contrast to the cause of a disease, does not explain why

the disease has developed, or why some individuals exposed to the risk factor do not become ill.

Logically it would seem that, if faced with a risk to health, individuals would consciously avoid that risk. Unfortunately, the process is not so simple, especially where an individual's primary perception of risk is associative rather than causative—or probabilistic rather than definitive. Furthermore, risk is a concept that pervades everyday life. Some element of risk is involved in almost all behaviour. For example, there is the risk of injury when crossing a busy street; the risk of loss of established relationships by forming new contacts; the risk of financial loss from an investment. Not only is some risk inevitable but also risk-taking behaviour provides intrinsic satisfaction to some individuals—for the challenge that it presents and the resulting 'high'. For many, life without risk would be like chilli without heat—edible but bland.

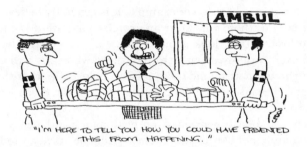

"I'M HERE TO TELL YOU HOW YOU COULD HAVE PREVENTED THIS FROM HAPPENING."

Some risks are considered acceptable, even where the actual risk is much higher than other risks that are considered unacceptable:

> People often willingly accept the risks of driving, calculated by risk assessors at one-in-a-hundred risk of death over a lifetime of driving. But the same people become outraged when a chemical plant or incinerator increases their risk of death by cancer, calculated by risk assessors at a one-in-a-million risk of death over a lifetime of exposure. (Covello 1995)

The past few decades of (frequently sensational) media reporting of each new study on risk factors for health and disease has left the general public rather confused and, in some cases, over-anxious that they might be in the category of a 'high-risk' group. As Lupton (1995) has observed: 'Individuals become defined and labelled by risk discourse, with diverse aspects of their lives ranging from their marital status to their choice of lunch becoming markers of risk.'

The focus of the present discussion is the risk of illness or death resulting from individual (psycho-behavioural) or external (socioenvironmental) causes. The determination of individual risk factors has become a major focus of secondary prevention programs. Risk factors for heart disease, for example, have been identified as:

- cigarette smoking
- hypertension
- hypercholesterolaemia
- high-fat diets
- inactivity
- obesity, and
- hereditary factors.

Risks for all the major lifestyle diseases have been similarly researched and listed with varying degrees of certainty. There is also a vast body of literature aimed at estimating the relative contributions of each of these factors to overall risk, and individuals have been divided into groups of high, medium and low risk, based on the presence or absence of such risk factors and their combinations. The underlying proposition is that by being informed of the existence of risk, high-risk individuals will be motivated to alter their lifestyle.

However, the likelihood of individuals being motivated to adopt health-enhancing types of behaviour—rather than those that are health-compromising (and therefore pose some risk to health)—is a function of the level of knowledge, attitudes and skills that the person possesses in relation to the health risk and the extent to which individual or socioenvironmental incentives or barriers (such as poverty) exist that facilitate or inhibit ceasing the risky behaviour.

Health knowledge and behaviour

It was a common belief among health professionals—and still is among some that knowledge about what influences health would be sufficient to motivate individuals towards healthy behaviour. However, the fact that knowledge is neither a necessary nor a sufficient condition for behaviour change is obvious from the fact that the deleterious aspects of smoking are almost universally known but about 22 per cent of the Australian population continues to smoke. Knowledge does not always motivate logically appropriate behaviour. Why?

First, individuals are bombarded with an enormous amount of information or 'clutter' in modern society. Each individual perceives this according to their own psychological predisposition. Individuals can select or ignore those things they don't wish to see or hear—because of anxiety or defences that have been built up to that message—and selectively focus on information that supports their existing beliefs and behaviour. For example a heavy smoker might go to the refrigerator during an anti-smoking television advertisement rather than face the anxiety that it might cause, and seize on any media reports that question the validity of the link between smoking and lung cancer.

Second, incoming information is interpreted in terms of personal experiences, background, beliefs, values and attitudes. For example, information about the link between smoking and lung cancer can be discounted by smokers who remind themselves of older smokers they know who 'lived to a ripe old age', by arguing that the link is 'only statistical', or by deluding themselves that 'if it was really that bad, the government would ban it'; in other words, by rationalising their actions.

Third, the input received and analysed must have personal relevance to the individual for action to be taken; that is, information that a particular diet has benefit for weight control is of little value to someone who does not want to lose weight, or who does not know someone who wants to lose weight.

Finally, even where an individual accepts that their behaviour puts them at risk, and has a full understanding of subsequent harms, other individual beliefs or environmental factors might inhibit adoption of healthy alternatives. A smoker might be experiencing a stressful period in his life and believe smoking is necessary to help him cope. A single father might believe that fast foods and sweets are nutritionally deficient and 'bad' for his children, but might prefer to give in to the child's demands rather than create conflict in the household. A woman might be convinced that 30 minutes of walking on most days would be beneficial to her health, but the neighbourhood is busy with traffic during the day, the area is poorly lit at night, and the footpaths are in poor condition anyway.

In summary, then ...

- In some cases, knowledge might be sufficient to elicit changes in behaviour, but in other cases, it might be neither necessary nor sufficient.
- Where knowledge is deemed important, this should be couched in terms relevant to the target audience.
- The transfer of knowledge into action is dependent on a wide range of internal and external factors, including attitudes and beliefs and the physical environment.
- For most individuals, the translation of knowledge into behaviour requires the development of specific skills (enabling factors), which could include interpersonal skills (e.g. parenting communication ability).

Attitudes, values and behaviour

To be acted on, knowledge needs to be incorporated by the individual in a way that both influences and is influenced by their personal attitudes and values with respect to health and health-enhancing behaviour. An individual's values affect a wide range of thought and behaviour patterns, in part by generating attitudes. Values precede attitudes in a manner that moves from the general to the specific; that is, a slim figure is prized by many in today's society, and this can predispose someone to act positively towards a weight-control program. Similarly, social justice and equity values can lead to positive attitudes towards specific programs targeting disadvantaged children or people with disabilities.

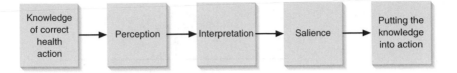

Figure 2.1: Phases between knowledge and behaviour
Adapted from Fishbein & Ajzen 1975

Bringing values and attitudes into the equation helps to explain the knowledge–action gap in many instances. Clearly, most people are at ease when the knowledge they hold is consistent with their attitudes and values. If discord arises (known as cognitive dissonance; discussed below), the facts are often interpreted (or misinterpreted) such that the contradiction between knowledge and attitudes is removed. Just as there is no clear association between knowledge and behaviour, there is no guaranteed clear progression from attitudes to behaviour. In most cases, attitude change precedes forming an intention to change, and thence behavioural change. In many cases, however, behaviour change could precede, and influence, attitudes. For example many people initially opposed to wearing seat belts became more favourable after the behaviour became compulsory; attitudes to drinking alcohol and driving changed after the introduction of random breath testing.

Maslow's Hierarchy of Needs

According to Maslow (1968), behaviour is motivated by a hierarchy of human needs (figure 2.2). At the base of this hierarchy is the desire to satisfy physiological needs: life's sustainers, such as food, water, oxygen and sleep. Once these are met, safety needs are next in the hierarchy, including the need for protection from harm and the alleviation of physical threat. Belongingness and love come next and, once these are satisfied, the need for self-esteem emerges as a primary motivator. Maslow's major contribution to health behaviour theory is his postulated highest level of needs, which is the desire for 'self-actualisation'. This reflects a desire to achieve the full capacity of one's ability and the self-satisfaction that accompanies it.

In practice, Maslow's theory clarifies for the health promotion practitioner why not everybody responds to the practitioner's 'obviously beneficial' and well-meaning interventions. For the low-income single parent, burdened with childcare responsibilities, and with little prospect of doing more than just 'coping' from day to day, the lure of a decrease in some forms of behaviour—which aid in the desire for belonging or identity (i.e. drinking alcohol or smoking tobacco)—for the promise of an intangible increase in health is hardly enticing. Health needs in this case might be compromised for the sake of satisfaction of lower-order needs before health promotion goals can be met.

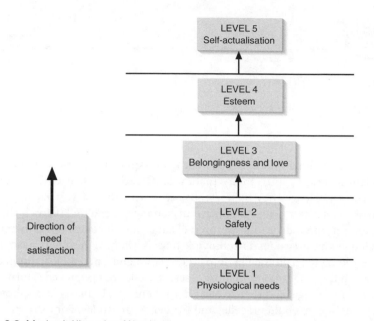

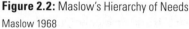

Figure 2.2: Maslow's Hierarchy of Needs
Maslow 1968

Models of individual behaviour change

An understanding of knowledge–attitude–behaviour models provides us with directions for setting communication objectives, and for generating message strategies and executions to achieve these objectives. These processes depend on a thorough understanding of the sorts of beliefs that influence attitudes towards the recommended healthy behaviour, how these beliefs and other facilitators and inhibitors influence intentions, and when and how intentions are fulfilled or not fulfilled.

Most of these models can be classified as 'attitude' models, whereby an attitude towards an object, person or form of behaviour is based on the set of beliefs held about that object, person or form of behaviour. For example, a person might believe that jogging:

- must be strenuous to be effective
- improves overall health, and
- increases alertness, but
- is liable to cause knee injuries.

Although this person might value an improvement in health and increased alertness, he might consider the consequence of injuries to be particularly traumatic. If positive beliefs outweigh negative beliefs, the attitude will be positive, and vice versa. This simple model assumes that all attributes have equal weighting. But this is generally not so. In the above example, a person with a knee injury might place far greater importance on this attribute than on the other attributes, and far greater importance than individuals who do not have any prior knee problems. That is, different individuals might have different importance ratings for the same attribute. Below, we describe several of the major models used in health promotion and the ways in which these have attempted to get around these problems.

The cognitive dissonance model

There have been several attitude theories based on the notion that people seek internal consistency between their beliefs, attitudes and behaviour, and that inconsistency is a psychologically uncomfortable state that leads to efforts to avoid or eliminate inconsistencies. The most influential of these theories has been that of Festinger's (1957) cognitive dissonance theory (CDT). CDT is concerned with the nature of the relations between various beliefs or 'cognitions'. Beliefs or cognitions might be:

* unrelated
* consistent (consonant), or
* inconsistent (dissonant; that is, in conflict).

For example, a belief that sexually transmitted chlamydial infection is a common disease, together with an intention to insist on condom use, are consonant beliefs; whereas a belief that smoking causes cancer, together with an intention to continue smoking, are dissonant beliefs.

The theory states that people will attempt to avoid dissonant experiences and that people experiencing dissonance will attempt to reduce it by changing their beliefs in a consonant direction. Efforts to reduce the dissonance will vary according to the degree of dissonance experienced. Mild dissonance might be ignored. The degree of dissonance will depend on the importance of the dissonance issue and the degree of disparity between the sets of dissonant cognitions; that is, dissonance is rarely experienced between just two cognitions, but rather between two sets of cognitions. As noted earlier, people generally hold a number of both negative and positive beliefs about health issues. A young smoker who believes that smoking is sophisticated, reduces anxiety and provides self-confidence in social situations, yet is harmful to health, smelly and expensive, might experience little dissonance because these two sets are relatively balanced. However, if cost has a greater degree of importance than the perceived benefits, then there will be a greater degree of dissonance.

Dissonance can be reduced in a number of ways:

* by adding new beliefs to one or other set
* by altering beliefs, or
* by altering the importance of the beliefs or the importance of the issue *per se.*

For example, adding beliefs that cigarette smoke contains toxic chemicals and that research by cigarette companies themselves confirms a link between smoking and cancer could move the above smoker into a dissonant state—resulting in attempts to quit to reduce the dissonance. Reducing the perceived likelihood of contracting a sexually transmitted disease will reduce the dissonance associated with a failure to use condoms. People who do not participate in physical activity, and who experience dissonance, might decide that the issue of exercise is simply not that important, and that other aspects of health—such as diet and relaxation—are far more important.

Many attempts to reduce dissonance are similar to what are termed cognitive defence mechanisms, or rationalisations. Credible sources such as celebrities or experts are sometimes used to create dissonance by having a trusted source (e.g. a popular footballer) deliver a message (smoking is 'uncool') that the target audience (young smokers) has previously rejected. The target is then faced with rejecting the trusted source, with accepting the previously rejected message, or with rationalising that the source is insincere in this regard ('he's being paid to say that!'). Another possible outcome is that the message is partly accepted and the source is simultaneously downgraded.

Dissonance theory also helps us understand selective attention and perception: avoiding messages that are inconsistent with one's beliefs avoids the uncomfortable state of dissonance, as does reinterpreting dissonant information in a way that is consonant with one's cognitions.

The dissonance model helps to explain why people act in ways that are often regarded as irrational and inconsistent.

The health belief model

The health belief model (Rosenstock 1974; see figure 2.3) is one of the oldest attempts to explain health behaviour. It was developed from work carried out in the 1950s, largely influenced by the works of the social psychologist Kurt Lewin. The principal tenet of the model is the way in which an individual perceives the world and how these perceptions motivate their behaviour. The model postulates that the readiness to take action for health stems from an individual's perception of their susceptibility to disease, its potential severity and the availability of an effective method for averting the disease. For example, mothers will insist on immunisation if they believe their child could contract a disease, the disease could have severe consequences, and immunisation could eliminate the danger.

Health-related action, then, is thought to depend on the simultaneous occurrence of three issues:

- whether the health issue is relevant
- whether the threat from it is regarded as important, and
- whether it's thought that doing something about it would reduce the threat.

INDIVIDUAL PERCEPTIONS   MODIFYING FACTORS   LIKELIHOOD OF ACTION

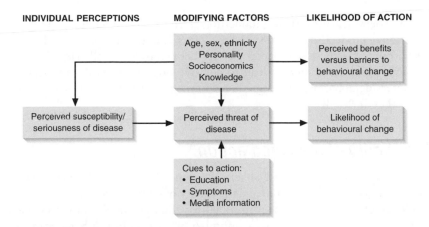

Figure 2.3: The health belief model
Adapted from Rosenstock 1974

More recently, the health belief model has been expanded to include the notion of 'self-efficacy', the belief that one has the ability to implement any change. Overall, then, for a behavioural change to succeed, individuals must have the incentive to change, feel threatened by their current behaviour, feel competent to implement a change and feel that a change will be beneficial at an acceptable cost.

The social learning theory model

Social learning theory was developed by Bandura (1977) and was perhaps the first theory of this type to introduce the notion of self-efficacy. Social learning theory is based on the belief that behaviour is determined by expectancies and incentives, in particular by expectancies about:

- environmental cues (i.e. beliefs about how events are linked and what leads to what)
- consequences of one's actions (i.e. how behaviour is likely to influence outcomes), and
- competency to perform the behaviour needed to influence outcomes (i.e. self-efficacy).

An incentive is defined as the value of a particular object or outcome. This might be health status, better looks or feeling better. Hence, for example, people who value changing their lifestyles to healthier behaviour will do so if they believe that:

- their current lifestyle poses a threat to any valued outcome (such as health or appearance)
- changes will reduce the threats, whether physical or psychological, and
- they are personally capable of adopting the new behaviour.

The social learning theory model forms the basis for 'edutainment': the inclusion of pro-health and pro-social messages in entertainment vehicles such as soap operas. In these soap operas, desired behaviour is modelled by admirable characters and are shown to lead to positive outcomes, while unattractive characters demonstrate undesired behaviour that leads to negative outcomes (Singhal et al. 2004).

The theory of reasoned action

The theory of reasoned action (Fishbein & Ajzen 1975)—and its later extensions, the theory of planned behaviour and the theory of trying—are perhaps the most developed of this type of model in social psychology and consumer decision making, and have been applied in a number of areas of health behaviour.

This approach proposes that behaviour is predicted by one's intention to perform the behaviour (how likely is it that you will take up a quit smoking program?). Intention, in turn, is a function of attitude towards that behaviour (e.g. do you feel that quitting is a good or bad idea?) and the perceived attitudes of friends, work colleagues and relatives to the behaviour (social norm) (e.g. do most people who are important to you think you should quit?). Attitude is a function of beliefs about the consequences of the behaviour (e.g. what are the outcomes of quitting?) weighted by an evaluation of the importance of each outcome (e.g. how important are these outcomes to you?). Social norm is a function of expectations of significant others (e.g. does your spouse, or a close friend think that you should quit?) weighted by the motivation to conform with each significant other (e.g. how important is it to do what your spouse, or that friend wants?).

The Fishbein and Ajzen model (figure 2.4) has two important features. First, there is a clear distinction between:

- attitudes towards objects, issues, events *per se*, and
- attitudes towards behaving in a certain way towards these objects, issues and events.

For example, an individual might have a favourable attitude towards Mercedes-Benz cars but a negative attitude towards actually buying one because this would involve borrowing a substantial amount of money at a high interest rate. Similarly, an individual might have a favourable attitude towards condoms *per se* but a negative attitude towards actually buying or carrying condoms. Hence, when exploring beliefs and attitudes to predict intentions and behaviour, it is necessary to be precise in terms of whether we are measuring attitudes towards an issue *per se* (e.g. exercise) or attitudes towards engaging in a certain form of behaviour (e.g. exercising). Furthermore, to predict intentions accurately, it is necessary to ensure that all relevant beliefs are uncovered. For example, it might be found that attitudes towards using condoms are favourable because only beliefs that were evaluated positively

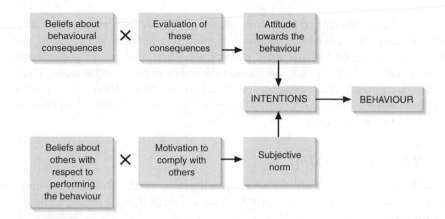

Figure 2.4: Theory of reasoned action

were included and beliefs that were evaluated negatively were unintentionally omitted. Formative (usually qualitative) research—based on group discussions or individual depth interviews—is often necessary to ensure that we are aware of all relevant beliefs that could contribute to an individual's overall attitude—and hence intentions.

Fishbein and Ajzen (1975) also distinguish between:

- the individual's beliefs related to the object or issues *per se,* and
- the individual's beliefs about what other people think about the issue— and how others think they should behave towards the issue (known as normative beliefs).

Hence, the Fishbein model incorporates social norms as an influence on attitudes and behaviour.

For example, an individual's attitude towards switching from a normal-strength beer to a reduced-alcohol beer will be a function of two components:

- their beliefs about the consequences of the behaviour (e.g. fewer hangovers, increased alertness, less risk of exceeding 0.05 per cent if breath-tested, less full-bodied taste), weighted by an evaluation of the beliefs (how positively or negatively the consequences—such as fewer hangovers, increased alertness and less taste—are viewed), and
- normative beliefs about how relevant others (i.e. friends, workmates and family) would view this form of behaviour (e.g. approve or disapprove), weighted by how important each of these relevant others is to the individual (e.g. workmates' opinions might be far more important than a spouse's opinion, or vice versa).

Again, it is necessary to ensure that all relevant beliefs of individuals, groups and populations are included in any measure of normative beliefs.

The theory of planned behaviour (Ajzen 1988) added a further component influencing intentions: the extent to which the individual perceives the behaviour to be under voluntary control, which is a function of perceived individual capabilities and environmental restrictions or facilitators. Thus, even where attitudes are positive and social norms are supportive, if someone believes adoption of a recommended form of behaviour is beyond their control, they are unlikely to do it.

The theory of trying

Building on Fishbein's theory of reasoned action in the field of consumer research, Bagozzi and Warshaw's (1990) theory of trying has two major elements of interest:

- It focuses on the individual's goals and separates trying to achieve these goals (i.e. attempting to quit smoking) from actual attainment of the goals (i.e. successfully quitting smoking). This is a far more realistic focus. For example, rather than attempting to determine the predictors of successful quitting, we should first determine the predictors of trying to quit.
- It introduces people's beliefs about the process of trying to adopt recommended behaviour and their attitudes towards success and failure. These are covered to some extent by other models; that is, in terms of costs involved in adopting recommended behaviour, but are conceptually clearer in the theory of trying.

Figure 2.5 shows that an individual's overall attitude towards trying to adopt some behaviour (e.g. reduced fat intake) to reach a goal (e.g. lose weight) is a function of three factors:

- the individual's attitude towards succeeding and perceived expectation of success
- the individual's attitude towards failing and perceived expectation of failing, and
- the individual's attitude towards the process of trying to lose weight.

Again, all of the above attitudes are based on various beliefs about consequences. These include beliefs about the consequences of successfully losing weight (e.g. feeling healthier), beliefs about the consequences of not losing weight (i.e. feeling depressed), beliefs about the process of actually losing weight (e.g. feeling hungry often), and the evaluation of these consequences.

An individual's intention to try to lose weight, then, will be determined by:

- their overall attitude towards trying to lose weight
- social norms about trying to lose weight (i.e. beliefs about relevant others' attitudes towards the individual losing weight), and
- the number of times the individual has tried to lose weight before.

Finally, actually trying to lose weight will be determined by:

- the individual's intention to try to lose weight
- the number of times the individual has tried to lose weight before, and
- the time since the last trial.

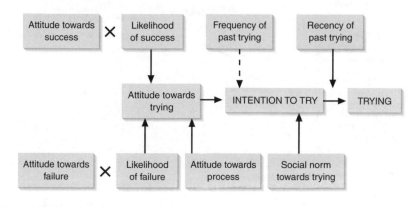

Figure 2.5: Theory of trying
Adapted from Bagozzi & Warshaw 1990

Protection motivation theory

Protection motivation theory (PMT) was developed by Rogers (1975), originally as a model of fear arousal to explain the motivational effect of fear or anxiety resulting from 'threat' communications. The theory assumes that people are motivated to protect themselves not only from physical threats but also from social and psychological threats (Rogers 1975, 1983).

PMT postulates four mental processes that appraise the presented health information, or threat, and that mediate attitudinal and behavioural change:

- the perceived severity of the threatened harmful event
- the perceived likelihood that the threatened outcome will occur (i.e. perceived vulnerability)
- the perceived effectiveness of the promoted 'healthy' alternative to avoid the occurrence of the threat (i.e. response efficacy), and
- the individual's self-perceived ability to perform the recommended 'healthy' alternative (i.e. self-efficacy).

These four processes result in two overall appraisals:

- an appraisal of the threat (based on the perceived severity and probability of occurrence), and
- a coping appraisal (based on the perceived response efficacy and self-efficacy).

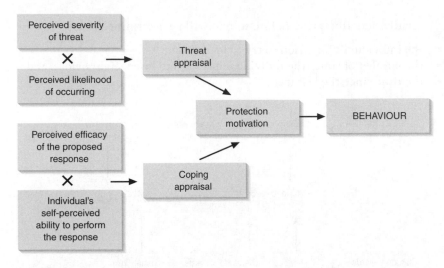

Figure 2.6: Protection-motivation theory

Given an appraisal that the threat is 'real' (i.e. personally relevant), and given an efficacious coping appraisal, an adaptive response is likely to occur. If the threat appraisal is discounted (e.g. by various defence mechanisms or rationalisations, such as 'it won't happen to me'), or the recommended alternative behaviour is not seen to be viable or effective (e.g. older smokers telling themselves the 'damage is already done' and hence 'quitting now won't help'), a maladaptive response is likely to occur (i.e. continuing to smoke or even increasing smoking).

The model emphasises the appraisal of threatening or supposedly fear-arousing communications. In its present form it does not allow for the assessment of messages that emphasise the positive effects or benefits of adopting the recommended behaviour. For example, both the positive benefits of exercising (e.g. enjoyment, social approval, mastery, alertness) and the avoidance of disadvantages by exercising (e.g. avoidance of heart disease) can be presented together, and often are (Donovan & Francas 1990). Hence, we need the additional mediating processes of the perceived attractiveness of the positive benefits to be gained by adopting the recommended behaviour, and the perceived efficacy of that behaviour to deliver those benefits.

Synthesising theories of health behaviour and developing practical programs

The main point to note from a presentation of these models is that communication campaigns must be carefully planned. Formative research helps to determine the various beliefs and perceptions that underlie attitudes, motivation and behaviour. Strategies can then be devised to:

1. change these beliefs (e.g. increase the perceived likelihood of a disease occurring)
2. change the evaluation of these beliefs (e.g. increase knowledge about the potential effects of this disease), or
3. introduce new beliefs (e.g. that having this disease increases susceptibility to an even more feared problem).

For practical purposes, the following are the key variables to research and incorporate in message strategies.

Consider an individual 'at risk' for heart disease:

1. What is the individual's perceived likelihood of contracting heart disease, given no change in their current behaviour?
    -   What beliefs or perceptions underlie this perceived likelihood?
    -   If the perceived likelihood is unrealistically low, what sort of information, presented in what way, and by whom, might increase this perceived likelihood?
2. What is the individual's perceived severity of heart disease? Is this realistic? If not, what sort of information, presented in what way and by whom, might change this perception?
3. What is the individual's attitude towards adopting the recommended alternative behaviour, such as a change in diet or adoption of exercise? Is some behaviour more acceptable than others? Why?
    -   What are the perceived benefits of continuing the risk behaviour?
    -   What are the perceived benefits and costs of the alternative behaviour?
    -   What social and physical barriers inhibit adoption of the recommended behaviour? What facilitators exist?
4. What is the individual's perceived likelihood of averting the threat if the recommended behaviour is adopted? If this is low, on what beliefs is this perception based? What information might change this perception?
5. What are the individual's beliefs about their ability to adopt the recommended behaviour? On what beliefs are these efficacy perceptions based? Is skills training required? What intermediate goals can be set to induce trial?
6. What appear to be the major motivations that would induce trial? Are positive benefits (e.g. feelings of wellness, increased capacity for physical activity) more motivating than negative benefits (e.g. avoidance of disease) for some individuals or groups, and vice versa for others?
7. What are the individual's main sources of information for health? Who are the major influencers? Who might be additional credible sources of information and influence?
8. How do social interactions, including the individual's extended family, club memberships, employment and home-care role, influence their health beliefs and behaviour?

9. Does the individual exhibit any personality characteristics that might inhibit or facilitate the adoption of healthy behaviour?
10. On a broader scale, how good is local doctors' knowledge of heart disease risk factors, and what is their willingness to undertake preventative measures with patients exhibiting these risk factors?
11. What factors exist in the individual's social, economic, work and physical environment that facilitate or inhibit physical activity and good eating habits?
12. To what extent do health bureaucrats understand heart disease risk factors, and what are their attitudes towards allocating funds to prevention?

Based on these models and the influence of environmental factors, behavioural scientists (e.g. Hill 2002; Fishbein et al. 1991; Elder et al. 1994), have generally agreed on a set of principles that guide the framework for interventions. Donovan and Henley (2003) list these as follows.

To perform a recommended behaviour, individuals must:

- have formed an intention to perform that behaviour, or made a (public) commitment to do so
- have no physical or structural constraints that prevent the behaviour being performed
- have the skills and equipment necessary to perform the behaviour
- perceive themselves as capable of performing the behaviour
- consider that the benefits of performing or not performing the behaviour outweigh the costs
- perceive the social pressure to perform the required behaviour as greater than that not to perform it
- perceive the behaviour to be consistent with their self-image, and
- perceive the behaviour to be consistent with their social roles.

Fishbein et al. (1991) consider that the first three of the above prerequisites are necessary and sufficient for behaviour to occur. Hence, if a violent man has formed a strong intention to call a helpline about his violence, if a telephone is easily accessible, and if the call can be made in private and with assured confidentiality, it is likely that the behaviour will occur. The remainder of the above variables primarily influence intention or facilitate/inhibit translating the intention into action.

The models described in this chapter apply equally to beliefs and attitudes about behaviour of interest as well as the beliefs and attitudes about the social and political issues related to that behaviour. Hence these models are useful not only for developing campaigns to promote healthy behaviour but also for developing advocacy campaigns. They form the basis for planning of health promotion campaigns, as considered in more detail in chapter 9.

> ## Career opportunities in health promotion
>
> Although a knowledge of theory alone does not usually justify vocational opportunities, the theoretical underpinnings of human health behaviour can lead to teaching opportunities in secondary and tertiary education, as well as in a number of vocational areas that require an understanding of a theoretical base. Theoretical knowledge is also a useful tool in commercial situations, such as the law, market research, advertising and consumer behaviour. Although not widely considered, a theoretical knowledge of behaviour also forms the basis of some occupations, such as politics, social service, sales and customer relations. In summary, a background in theory is almost a prerequisite for any form of career in practice that involves understanding the behaviour of other people.

References

Ajzen, I., 1988, *Attitudes, Personality, and Behaviour*, Dorsey Press, Chicago.

Ajzen, I., & Fishbein, M., 1980, *Understanding Attitudes and Predicting Social Behaviour*, Prentice Hall, Englewood Cliffs, NJ.

Bagozzi, R. P., & Warshaw, P. R., 1990, 'Trying to consume', *J Consum Res* 17:127–40.

Bandura, A., 1977, *Social Learning Theory*, Prentice Hall, Englewood Cliffs, NJ.

Covello, V., 1995, 'Risk perception and communication', *Can J Pub Health* 86(2):78–82.

Donovan, R. J., & Francas, M., 1990, 'Understanding communication and motivation strategies', *Aust Health Rev* 10:103–14.

Donovan, R. J., & Henley, N., 2003, *Social Marketing: Principles and Practice*, IP Communications, Melbourne.

Elder, J. P., Geller, E. S., Hovell, M. F., & Mayer, J. A., 1994, *Motivating Health Behaviour*, Delmar, NY.

Festinger, L. A., 1957, *A Theory of Cognitive Dissonance*, Stanford University Press, Palo Alto, Calif.

Fishbein, M., & Ajzen, I., 1975, *Beliefs, Attitudes, Intention and Behavior: An Introduction to Theory and Research*, Addison-Wesley, Boston, Mass.

Fishbein, M., Middlestadt S., & Hitchcock, P. J., 1991, 'Using information to change sexually transmitted disease-related behaviours: an analysis based on the theory of reasoned action', in Wasserheit, J. N., Aral, S. O., Holmes, K. K. (eds), *Research Issues in Human Behavior and Sexually Transmitted Diseases in the AIDS Era*, American Society for Micro-Biology, Washington DC.

Harper, A. C., Holman, C. D. J., & Dawes, V. P., 1994, *The Health of Populations: An Introduction* (2nd edn), Churchill Livingstone, Melbourne.

Hill, D., 2002, 'Cancer prevention: asking the hard questions', paper presented to the State Cancer Conference, Perth, WA.

Lee, C., & Owen, N., 1986, 'Use of psychological theories on understanding the adoption and maintenance of exercising', *Aust J Sc Med Sport*, 18(2):22–5.

Lupton, D., 1995, *The Imperative of Health: Public Health and the Regulated Body*, Sage, London.

Maslow, A. H., 1968, *Towards a Psychology of Being*, Van Nostrand, NY.

Nutbeam, D., & Harris, H., 2004, *Theory in a Nutshell: A Practical Guide to Health Promotion Theories* (2nd edn), McGraw-Hill, Sydney.

Rogers, R. W., 1975, 'A protection motivation theory of fear appeals and attitude change', *J Psych* 91:93–114.

—— 1983, 'Cognitive and physiological process in fear appeals and attitude change: a revised theory of protection motivation', in Cacioppo, J., & Petty, R. (eds), *Social Psychophysiology*, Guilford Press, New York.

Rosenstock, I. M., 1974, 'Historical models of the health belief model', in Becker, M. H. (ed.), *The Health Belief Model and Personal Health Behavior*, Charles B. Slack, Thorofare, NJ.

Singhal, A., Cody, M. J., Rogers, E., & Sabido, M., 2004, *Entertainment-Education and Social Change*, Lawrence Erlbaum Associates, Mahwah, NJ.

Chapter 3
Focus on the individual

Summary of main points

- Health promotion began as health education, with an individual focus in parental and clinical situations.
- Individual approaches in clinical settings are usually, but not always, associated with secondary or tertiary prevention.
- Most individual approaches involve some form of one-to-one counselling, for which outcomes can be improved by using special techniques, such as motivational interviewing.
- Primary health care in future will be expected to incorporate a much bigger role in health promotion.
- New technology, such as the Internet, offers unique opportunities for access to individual information.
- New opportunities exist for health promotion professionals to work at a clinical (one-to-one) level, dealing particularly with lifestyle and chronic diseases.

Why individual approaches?

An individual focus has been the cradle of health promotion. It began as health education, with an individual focus on a one-to-one basis: mother to child, then later midwife to mother and doctor to patient. The influence of a credible personal source of health information remains strong and should not be undervalued, although a number of factors have changed the emphasis on this in recent times:

- With large populations, the intended audience is so numerous that it is too labour-intensive to reach everyone in this manner. In a traditional village, with extended families and a close interpersonal communication network, an individual focus might have been plausible. In a modern industrialised society, not only is it difficult to gain access to people but also health information is competing with a myriad of other messages, often from anti-health forces.

- Most information concerning health is now so technical and complex that a 'translation' process is necessary to transform scientific and medical terminology into information that can be understood and acted on by the general public.
- The advent of the Internet has meant that easy access to wide-ranging health information is now available at the click of a mouse. This makes information transmission much quicker and easier (although the reliability of some health information accessed on the Internet could be questionable).

Although an individual health promotion practitioner, even in a small community, would face a daunting task in counselling each individual in that community, there are many opportunities to reach individuals through other means; for example, enlisting various professionals who deal with people on a personal basis to incorporate health promotion into their role. In this way, the health promotion practitioner could facilitate the health promotion role of other health professionals. For example an estimated 80 per cent of people visit a general practitioner (GP) as their first reference for health matters, and many regard their GP as their most influential source of information. There is therefore potential for involving the GP in health promotion. With the changing nature of disease, there has also been a rise in new health practitioners, such as lifestyle counsellors, life coaches, personal trainers, practice nurses and weight loss specialists, to help deal with contemporary health problems, particularly chronic diseases and their risk factors.

Individual methods in health promotion have limitations, particularly time and cost-effectiveness. However, the interactive nature of face-to-face communication allows greater possibilities for personal influence and potential lifestyle change than perhaps any other communication medium.

Individual methods

One of the most common individual methods in prevention is that which is generally referred to as 'patient education'. This reflects the fact that individual methods of health promotion are usually, but not exclusively, associated with either secondary prevention (i.e. attempts to reverse the early symptoms of disease) or tertiary prevention (i.e. attempts to slow the progress of a disease that already exists, such as after a heart attack).

On the other hand, individual risk factor assessment and identification can be regarded as secondary prevention (where illness risks are identified) or primary prevention (intervention aimed at avoiding illness before any disease state or symptoms exist). The common and important problem of hypertension (high blood pressure) offers a good example of primary, secondary and tertiary prevention:

- Primary prevention is education about avoiding obesity and inactivity, which can lead to hypertension.
- Secondary prevention is the detection and treatment of high blood pressure so as to avoid heart disease or stroke.
- Tertiary prevention is action, including medication, to prevent recurrence of a stroke or heart attack (in this case associated with hypertension). This can include rehabilitation after such events.

One-to-one individual methods are not as appropriate in the area of primary prevention, because of the cost incurred in reaching individuals in large populations, many of whom might never develop the specific disease. For this situation, group and whole population approaches, aimed at making small health gains across larger populations, are more suitable. These will be discussed in chapter 4.

Patient education

Philosophy

Patient education can be classified according to who delivers the education (e.g. nurses, doctors, community health workers), the type of ailment involved (e.g. diabetes, heart disease, cancer), the intended audience (e.g. the elderly, mothers, mothers-to-be), where the education is delivered (e.g. hospital, medical or allied health professional settings) or the type of educational process (e.g. programmed learning, self-care, distance education). The primary philosophy is that patient education should:

- be integrated into patient care
- be developed in conjunction with patients
- involve interdisciplinary involvement, and
- have specific and measurable goals.

In addition, patient education programs should involve families, partners and friends, as well as the patients themselves. The discussion below is categorised into settings in which patient education can occur. For more detailed information on patient education readers are referred to the work of Redman (2001), Lorig (2000) or Falvo (2004).

Hospital settings

The historical role of hospital involvement in health promotion goes back to the beginnings of health care. As knowledge about the causes of disease increased, it became incumbent upon hospitals to try to reduce illness through programs aimed at the root causes of these illnesses. Initially, only first-aid classes were offered, but these have expanded to include many types of programs at both the inpatient and outpatient levels. Modern developments in this area include the Budapest Declaration on health-promoting hospitals, which contains a framework for implementing the aims of the Ottawa Charter for Health Promotion in the hospital setting (WHO 1991).

Inpatient programs

Hospital inpatient programs are based on the premise that patients have a right to know not only the current status of their health but also what they can do to improve it and to prevent recurrences of illness. Inpatient programs can include:

- provision of appropriate health information
- a brief intervention by a health professional with an inpatient who presents with risk factors, or
- a specific intervention, such as a nurse-facilitated smoking-cessation program in surgical pre-admission clinics (Haddock & Burrows 1997).

Inpatient programs can include general health education material (e.g. maintaining a healthy lifestyle) or education for specific ailments (e.g. diabetes, asthma, heart disease). These programs can include audiovisual resources, lecture, discussions, one-to-one counselling and printed materials, such as brochures and pamphlets. Depending on the client group, multilingual services might be required, in which case the health promotion practitioner could act as a coordinator of services rather than a deliverer. Media skills can be useful to develop audiovisual material, which might be specific to a particular inpatient situation or available for more general use. Multimedia resources are now also available commercially. Hospital libraries might hold many of these for loans.

Hospital staff support for health promotion activities with patients is generally high, particularly in the more commonly seen areas of smoking cessation and skin cancer prevention. However, sufficient funding, support from relevant personnel and availability of resources and training appear to be barriers to more hospital-based health promotion activities being undertaken (Anderson et al. 1995).

The role of the health promotion practitioner in patient education includes the following:

- identifying the health problems that are amenable to education intervention
- formulating patient education goals and policies
- planning a course of action appropriate to these needs and goals
- determining the health behaviour and actions of patients that contributed to their specific health problems
- evaluating the education interventions to see whether they made a difference to a patient's health status

- planning staff development programs for health providers and other members of the health team on learning strategies and methods, and
- helping select, prepare and distribute educational materials to be used in patient education programs.

Resources of hospitals and clinics have historically been barely sufficient to allow them to carry out the curative and palliative care that the public demands. In this context, the diversion of resources or allocation of additional funding to the area of health promotion might sometimes be greeted less than enthusiastically by hospital and medical administrators. However, the opportunity of reaching a 'captive' audience—with a vested interest in avoiding a recurrence of their illness—is one that offers challenges for the health promotion practitioner. Not the least of these is the problem of patient adherence to preventive practices once the patient has returned to their normal life (see case study 3.1).

Case study 3.1

Nurse–patient effects on diabetes management

Lack of compliance with diabetes advice and prescription is a common problem, and complications often develop quickly. Researchers in the Netherlands tested adherence to a set of guidelines proposed for diabetes care in the hospital setting when these were imparted by doctors, nurses or other hospital staff. Compliance was greatest when a specialist diabetic nurse was used for patient education, which suggests that the selection of health promotion personnel could be just as important as the information imparted, if not more important. Specialist nurses obviously have the skills and time to ensure greater compliance with the message than other health personnel.

Dijkstra et al. 2004

Outpatient settings

Outpatient visits to hospitals outnumber inpatient experiences by a factor of approximately 10 to 1. Non-hospital care is likely to increase even further with current economic pressure on health-care funding and the consequent move to alternative health-care settings and arrangements, such as day surgeries, short-stay clinics and health-maintenance organisations (HMOs). Therefore outpatient services represent a useful mode of health promotion intervention.

Outpatient services are frequently used by the elderly and the disadvantaged, as well as by many who don't necessarily use clinical care as much as social services and who, by using these services, overload their capacity and restrict availability to those more in need. Because they are often frequented by clients from disadvantaged groups, they can also be a setting for addressing social needs of individuals and possibly their neighbourhoods.

A number of factors need to be taken into consideration in planning health promotion programs for outpatient facilities. These include:

- the characteristics of the outpatient staff (number, type, cooperation, time availability)
- the characteristics of the outpatient population (readiness to learn, number, type)
- the contact time of staff and patients
- availability of space, and
- availability and appropriateness of resources (e.g. audiovisual equipment).

Inpatient and outpatient programs should be complementary. Hence the latter might also involve:

- the use of multimedia resources
- the introduction of inpatient information needed to assist discharge and recovery
- printed materials with information on general and specific needs and
- advice to and training of staff for basic outpatient counselling and delivery of educational kiosks.

Because patient involvement could be high in relation to messages that relate directly and immediately to their own health outcomes, outpatient departments can make use of on-the-spot educational materials such as pamphlets, educational videos and user-friendly computer programs and interactive kiosks.

Group programs can also be run in both the inpatient and the outpatient setting. Group classes, support sessions, community seminars and health fairs are all methods that have been tried with varying degrees of success. Examples of health problems addressed by patient education programs include diabetes, asthma, heart disease, stroke, obesity and mental illness.

Self-care and self-management education

Patient education can assist individuals to become more effective in self-management, particularly in the case of chronic disease, thereby reducing costly demands on health services. The movement for self-care began in the 1970s. However, it was not initially integrated into organised medical care programs. More recently a systematised approach has been taken to reintegrate self-care into the health system.

Arthritis self-management programs, for example, are now integrated into many clinical practices' guidelines and policies, and have become the core business of many arthritis foundations. These involve educational programs designed to empower individuals to promote health and prevent adverse sequelae from their disease, as well as teach them how to interact effectively with the health system, monitor their physical and emotional status and make appropriate management decisions on the basis of the results of self-monitoring (Osborne, Spinks & Wicks 2004).

Self-management concentrates on three main tasks (medical, role and emotional management) and six main skills (problem solving, decision making, resource utilisation, the formation of a patient–provider partnership, action planning and self tailoring). The mechanism through which this has been evaluated as having a positive effect on health outcomes is by improving self-efficacy in the patient (Lorig & Holman 2003; Lorig 2000).

Counselling, brief interventions and motivational interviewing

Counselling is a form of systematic guidance offered by health professionals in which a person's problems are discussed and advice given. Most of the methods discussed here involve some form of counselling, and counselling can include a range of different principles and techniques. Brief interventions are a form of counselling aimed at making the most of any opportunity to raise awareness, share information and get a person thinking about making changes to their health-related behaviour. A clinician seeing a patient for an unrelated matter, for example, might note that the patient has gained significant weight or has taken up smoking since a previous visit, and then proceed to raise awareness about the related health risks and offer advice for dealing with them.

Motivational interviewing is a process of questioning that can be used effectively in counselling to raise a patient's likelihood of complying with a clinician's prescription. Motivational interviewing has a structured format that can be taught to clinicians and other health professionals (Rollnick, Heather & Bell 1992).

Case study 3.2

Targeting behaviour change

Scottish exercise researcher Alison Kirk used motivational interviewing to target messages for diabetes patients identified as being in one of the first three levels of 'stages of change' (see chapter 5) to become more physically active. A control group were given only standard advice on treatment for their disease. After six months the targeted group had not only considerably increased their level of physical activity as measured by movement sensors but had also increased their fitness, reduced their blood sugars and improved their blood lipids. They had also shifted along the 'stages of change' in line with an improvement in motivation.

Kirk et al. 2003

Primary health care

'Primary health care' refers to policies formalised in the Declaration of Alma Ata in 1978 and subsequently adopted by the WHO and other UN organisations. Primary health care is concerned with the first level of the health system, the initial point of contact for people seeking assistance with a health problem or for general health-related advice. As this level of service requires structures to integrate with each other and the whole health system, primary health care is also an approach to service delivery.

The primary health-care approach comprises a set of principles, including:

- intersectoral collaboration
- coordination of primary, secondary and tertiary health services to facilitate continuity of care
- balanced resource use addressing both intermediate needs and longer-term issues
- a population focus, with special attention to high-risk and vulnerable groups as a precondition for equity in health outcomes and health-care access, and
- appropriate technology (WHO 1983).

As a signatory to this global policy direction, Australia has seen this commitment articulated in state and national health policies. These policy initiatives have led to the growth of primary health-care centres and the establishment of university-based centres of excellence in primary health care.

Health promotion is a key strategy of primary health-care practitioners, particularly through:

- health promotion planning that facilitates community involvement in the identification of priorities and the ownership of programs
- the provision of intersectoral advocacy for healthy public policy, and
- the delivery of interactive health education.

Although it is important that primary health care is adopted within secondary and tertiary health-care settings, the community health services sector provides the leading edge for implementation of primary health care owing mainly to their collaboration in defined localities or neighbourhoods. Other groups to be considered under this heading are doctors and allied health workers and pharmacists.

Community health centres

Within any community, community health services combine health promotion, early detection and intervention, rehabilitation and the management of chronic health problems. Established in Australia in the 1970s, community health centres—providing accessible, primary health care in a user-friendly, multipurpose setting—are logical venues for all levels of preventive intervention in both individual and group settings. The health centre can also be a venue for community development action, which stimulates programs from the ground up.

Community health centres are often the source of much health information material and/or have access to central library facilities. Individual counselling, risk factor assessment and audiovisual education can be carried out in the health centre setting, including programs covering:

- relationship counselling, maternal and child health, crisis counselling
- psychological assessments and early interventions
- chronic disease care, and
- care coordination and counselling.

Case study 3.3

Focusing on mothers

Historically, prenatal care and health promotion has been concerned with delivering a good birth outcome (such as ideal birth weight) for the infant. This was (rightly) aimed at reducing the high rates of infant mortality associated with early and pre-developed societies. However, while infant mortality rates have improved dramatically, at least in non-indigenous populations, there has been a shift of focus away from the health of the mother, resulting in big increases in gestational diabetes mellitus (GDM), which can progress to later type 2 diabetes. In Pacific island cultures in particular, adoption of European approaches to childbirth has meant a significant decrease in activity levels of new mothers and an excessive fat gain as they are 'wrapped in cotton-wool' by relatives to ensure a good birth outcome.

Recent attention has therefore been given to exercise and diet programs in pregnancy, with the goal of remaining active and not gaining excessive weight. Because of the value of exercise in maintaining blood sugar levels, innovative programs using aerobics, aquarobics and resistance training are now being promoted. Research on resistance training using rubber bands has shown a decrease in the effects of GDM from twenty-six to thirty-two weeks of pregnancy compared with a standard recommended diet program. This, and other recent work showing the reversibility of early stage type 2 diabetes with lifestyle change, is likely to change the nature of antenatal health promotion in the future. Marriage and pregnancy in island and indigenous cultures offer ideal opportunities for focusing pre- and post-natal health promotion messages aimed at ensuring the health of the mother, as well as the baby.

Brankston et al. 2004

Medical and allied professional programs

These programs consist of patient education services provided by doctors, dentists, physiotherapists, dietitians, podiatrists, occupational therapists and other health professionals. Because time is often limited, the most effective vehicle for health promotion is a brief intervention supported by relevant resources and information.

General medical practice

General medical practice is the first point of contact with the health-care system for the majority of people in Australia. More than 82 per cent of the population visit a GP at least once a year and, on average, people visit a GP approximately five times each year (Britt et al. 2004). It is estimated that up to 60 per cent of attendances at general practice are precipitated by a lifestyle-based—and hence predominantly preventable—cause (AIHW 2004). However, problems within the medical profession, and various political and social trends, have been documented as impeding the ability of general practice to realise its full potential in the Australian health-care system.

The General Practice Strategy introduced by the Australian Government in 1992 aimed to improve access to general practice services, encourage the improved integration of general practice with the rest of the health-care system, enhance the quality and cost-effectiveness of general practice, and support training for GPs (DHSH 1996). The strategy included the establishment of networks of GPs, linked for the purpose of reducing the sense of professional isolation experienced by GPs, who are often excluded from involvement in hospital care, teaching, research and local or regional health planning. These networks—known as Divisions of General Practice—provide infrastructure and funding that enable GPs to undertake cooperative activities to improve their integration with other elements of the health system. Key roles identified for such networks/organisations were 'health promotion, illness prevention and population health activities at the local level, including coordination of general practitioners' participation in regional and national programs' (General Practice Consultative Committee 1992).

In line with international trends to address equity in health outcomes in Western countries, special funding has been provided to make GP health promotion and other activities a reality. This finance will encourage population-based planning, which identifies long-term goals and specific target areas in which maximum health gains can be achieved. Such health priority areas for GP divisional work include: vaccine-preventable infectious diseases; chronic disease prevention and management (such as diabetes, arthritis and asthma); cardiovascular disease; injury; mental health; cancer; and particular population groups, such as children and Aboriginal and Torres Strait Islander people.

General medical practice continues to provide an important and cost-effective setting for health promotion because of the high patient-contact rates and the perceived credibility of GPs by the public. For example smoking-intervention programs based on GPs have resulted in significant reduction in smoking (Richards et al. 2003). The majority of patients considered that their chances of success were greater if a doctor administered the smoking-intervention programs, and that having the results of lung-function and blood tests (explained in relation to the risks of cardiovascular and respiratory diseases) constituted a strong incentive to stop smoking. As well as encouraging smoking-cessation, GP patient education has demonstrated success with many other health problems, including HIV/AIDS (Gallagher 1989), back pain (Roland & Dixon 1989), hypertension (Watkins et al. 1987) and the reduction of excessive alcohol consumption (Wallace, Cutler & Haines 1988; Richmond et al. 1998).

In a study of GP attitudes and use of patient education resources, Roche, Bennetts and Mira (1994) found that, although time constraints limit patient education opportunities, the use of health education literature is still identified as an efficient way to partially overcome this problem. In this study pamphlets and tear-off sheets were the most commonly used materials. Doctors had a strong preference for materials to be available in a greater range of health areas and for them to be simple in design.

Nevertheless, because of a range of barriers restricting them, it would appear that doctors could still be under-utilised in performing a community-based health education role outside their clinical practice, despite their willingness to participate (Bonevski, Sanson-Fisher & Campbell 1996). Among these barriers is a lack of confidence by GPs owing to inadequate training in, and information on, health promotion (Girgis & Sanson-Fisher 1996). The need for this kind of training is being addressed by Divisions of General Practice in partnership with health promotion practitioners. For example nearly 5000 general practitioners in Australia, New Zealand and the South Pacific had completed at least one stage of a Post-Graduate Medical Certificate in Weight Control and Obesity Management coordinated by one of the authors (GE) by mid-2004 (Egger & Thorburn in press).

Because clinical health professionals do have limitations on knowledge in health promotion, the possibility of expert visits to such people, much in the manner of drug detailers, could be yet another method of getting information to the public. Exercise, stress management and drug education are areas in which health professionals accept their educational limitations and, in some cases, welcome expert advice. Health promotion practitioners could consider using the increasing interest shown by the pharmaceutical industry in funding conferences or professional 'update' seminars for health-care professionals as a vehicle for providing training in patient education on a range of health issues (Gruber et al. 1997).

Allied health professionals

A number of new disciplines now exist to aid health promotion at the clinical level. In addition to traditional disciplines such as dietitians, psychologists, podiatrists, physiotherapists and so on, new disciplines include practice nurses within medical surgeries, lifestyle counsellors, life coaches and personal trainers. Under new government policy for utilising allied health professionals introduced in 2004, personnel trained in these areas will be able to work in an integrated clinical team alongside general practitioners to provide lifestyle programming to patients with metabolic and lifestyle-related disorders, such as obesity, diabetes and heart disease. This offers new career opportunities in health promotion for those who might choose to work at the clinical (one-on-one) level rather than at the population level.

Pharmacies

The potential of pharmacies as health promotion outlets is only beginning to be realised. In some states, health insurance companies are utilising pharmacies as an outlet for summary information sheets, which also advertise the company's services. As shelf space is a priority in pharmacies, special pamphlet racks are provided by the companies.

A pharmacy fact sheet program—the Pharmacy Self-Care Fact Cards—and self-help touch service computer programs were developed by the Pharmaceutical Society of Australia as part of their Pharmacy Self-Care Program.

Pharmacies are also becoming involved in risk-factor screening for such problems as osteoporosis (Goode, Swiger & Bluml 2004), smoking cessation (Sinclair, Bond & Stead 2004) and other forms of health promotion (Chandra, Malcolm & Fetters 2004). They are increasingly being used as a primary care service system (Carmichael et al. 2004).

Home health-care providers

With growing concern about hospital costs and an increasingly ageing population, there is increasing demand for home-based health care. Usually these services come from the ranks of nursing and are employed by government, local hospitals or community and non-governmental organisations (e.g. Blue Care, Silver Chain). However, there is an increasing trend towards privately run home-care services.

Case study 3.4

The health promoting pharmacy

Trials are being undertaken to test shelf spaces in pharmacies devoted to lifestyle-based health problems, such as weight control, quitting smoking and heart disease. This accords with research showing that pharmacists can be effective in weight control management with customers (Ahrens, Hower & Best 2003). This will mean a shift to pharmacists (and assistants) offering health services, not just products and advice, and hence they might require extra training along the lines of chronic disease management.

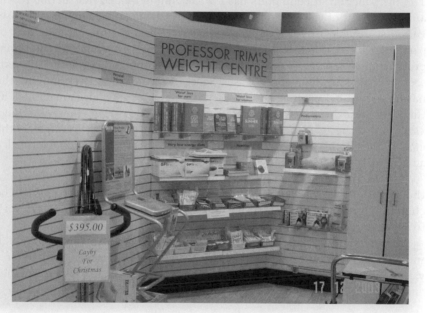

The opportunity for home-care patient education is thus likely to increase. This is likely to be aimed mainly at seniors and, to a lesser extent, at people with a disability. Areas for development include nutrition, exercise, prevention of trauma, and other aspects of self-care, such as preventing falls. Intervention could consist of written and audiovisual material, but is more likely to be in the form of one-to-one counselling. The health promotion practitioner in these settings could act as a trainer of the home-care provider in health promotion skills.

The increasing use of information and communications technology in health has also signalled a potential expansion of home care with home monitoring of vital signs for patients with chronic disease. Home visits by nurses in person can be replaced by telemedicine videophone consultations (Celler, Lovell & Basilakis 2003).

Programmed learning, self-help materials and the Internet

'Programmed learning' refers to learning carried out in a sequential pattern. It is generally computer-based or by means of written, structured manuals, and is often used for individualised education and change, particularly for patient education and professional-training programs.

Internet

The introduction of computers has led to computer-aided instruction (CAI), and the advent of the Internet has made it available at the click of a mouse. Patients are able to get readily available, free information about areas of particular interest just by following search engines, thus placing additional pressure on medical practitioners, for whom one topic is only a small area of their knowledge base. Easier access to information is changing the nature of medical practice and necessitating greater specialty areas, such as the allied health professionals referred to above. However, there is a huge variation in the relevance and quality of Internet sites. For example in the area of weight loss, probably less than 5 per cent provide reliable health advice (Miles et al. 2000).

Also, despite the wide proliferation of services, there is little evidence of the effects of the Internet on health-care outcomes (Bessell et al. 2002). The challenge is to equip consumers with the knowledge and discriminatory skill to appraise the available information selectively.

New technology has led to the development by health professionals of interactive computer games to increase skill and self-efficacy for patients in a variety of health-related issues, including illicit drug use, use of performance enhancing drugs, and safe-sex negotiation (Thomas, Cahill & Santilli 1997).

Email

Email has opened up opportunities for delivering information to large numbers of individuals at the click of a mouse. Previously this required printing, layout, publishing and postage of materials, all of which is costly and timely. Email, however, allows distribution to be done simply and cheaply. Hence groups defined by certain interest areas can receive regular newsletters, updates, journal articles or other forms of support from an authoritative source. Email is also suggested as a possible way of the future for medical practice to involve patients in their own care and optimise face-to-face visits (Meyer 2004).

Programmed learning and distance learning health programs

Programmed learning works best when health promotion practitioners have the resources to produce their own educational modules and materials for a specific market. Consumer preferences indicate that programmed learning in the form of distance learning programs might be more desirable than face-to-face formats for some people, particularly more highly educated and higher-income groups (Sherwood et al. 1998). Programs can range from being totally self-help with minimal contact to adding a component to a shared care program. They have also been offered at no cost, at commercial rates or with different forms of cost incentive. Reported success rates are generally higher with some level of payment, perhaps indicating a level of self-selection through commitment.

Programmed instruction requires frequent use of materials and situations that are more appropriate for an individual approach rather than a group situation (e.g. in cases of geographical isolation or sensitivity). The use of programmed learning for quit smoking and exercise instruction, for example, has been developed and evaluated in South Australia by Owen (1988). 'GutBusters'—the first major men's 'waist-control' program, developed in Australia in 1991—provided programmed material on a commercial basis for up to 10 000 individual men a year. Evaluation of the program showed it to be more effective than group-based weight-control initiatives (Egger et al. 1996).

Programmed learning is most appropriate when:

- the range of individual differences is great enough to require individual learning
- the topic is sensitive and calls for a degree of privacy (e.g. sexually transmitted diseases)
- the subject material is straightforward and does not require clarification, and
- there are sufficient funds and support to ensure continuity of such a program.

Australia offers particular challenges for health promotion in the area of programmed learning because of the existence of rural and isolated people with specific health needs.

Shared care

Shared care has been used as an effective delivery option for many health-related programs ranging from pregnancy to aged care. Because most health problems these days call for multidisciplinary input, the idea of shared care between disciplines is a logical approach to service delivery. This strategy has been successfully used in the management of a number of conditions, including diabetes, mental health, drug abuse, antenatal care, prostate cancer, AIDS, cardiovascular disease and depression (Hickman et al. 1994).

Options that optimise use of the practitioner's time by combining consultations with developed programs and distance-learning courses might be a logical direction for the future. Changes in the health system to allow care planning and case conferencing with allied health professionals also make this a more viable option for primary carers.

Case study 3.5

Packaged shared care for weight loss

'Professor Trim's Medically Supervised Weight Loss Programs' (Male and Female) were developed as a follow-on from the GutBusters (Men's Waist Loss) Program of the 1990s. Professor Trim's packs contain CDs, workbooks, a textbook, a pedometer, stress measures, links to the Internet (www. professortrim.com) and links with a trained GP or personal weight coach. The package is designed to provide information on weight control to literate patients, thus saving clinicians having to go over the basics repetitively with each new patient.

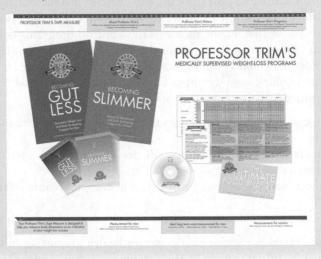

Egger, Stanton & Cameron-Smith 2002

Health promotion shopfronts

Shopfront services for health promotion materials and programs have been tried in various cities (in the city centre or in major shopping malls) around the country. Although these are community-based, the strategy is focused on large numbers of one-to-one interactions.

The first test of health promotion shopfronts was as part of the experimental North Coast Healthy Lifestyle program in 1978–81 in Lismore, NSW (Egger et al. 1983). Since then, shopfronts of various forms have been created throughout Australia, including those for non-government organisations, such as the National Heart Foundation, cancer councils and Diabetes Australia. Shopfronts are able to provide many of the services available in all forms of health promotion: literature, risk factor assessment, counselling, lectures, group programs, and computerised instruction and testing. Their major advantage is that they 'get in people's way', often while they are shopping, and so they can reach such groups as blue-collar workers or mothers who might not seek health information and programs in formal health-care settings or government offices. Shopfronts could also be a source of funds for an organisation, although commercial lease costs in central public access points, such as city malls and shopping centres, could be prohibitive.

The shopfront can be used as a source of two-way interaction in the health promotion process with clients contributing experiences and needs to staff, and programs being developed to cater for those needs. A shopfront can serve as a community focus for large-scale health promotion programs and campaigns and become a staging point for promotions as well as a reference point for materials and information.

Because of the issues of cost and sustainability, health promotion shopfronts—pioneered by state and territory health departments in the 1970s and 1980s—are today more likely to be found within the operations of private-sector health insurance organisations and/or pharmacies.

Risk factor assessments

As noted in the introduction to this chapter, risk factor assessment is usually used as a means of secondary prevention. However, in some cases (e.g. nutrition analysis, fitness assessment, body weight analysis) it can be used in primary prevention to develop programs that could enable an individual to stay healthy. A number of risk factor assessments is currently available, and the form and source of some of these are listed below. Risk factor measurements can be carried out directly by an experienced health promotion practitioner; alternatively, the practitioner could facilitate assessments by other qualified health professionals.

Health risk appraisal (HRA)

Health risk appraisals are available through a number of computerised tests that are often accessible via shopfront services or existing health-related outlets, such as pharmacies.

HRAs have limited validity because of the subjective nature of many of the questions. However, a study of the accuracy of HRAs in predicting mortality has shown that they could be appropriate for identifying high-risk populations for health interventions (Faxman & Eddington 1987). They could also serve as a motivational starting point for some individuals by creating a perceived need for behaviour change.

Blood chemistry screening

Recent developments in blood chemistry have broadened the range of measures available for assessing risk (see box 'Risk measurements for the overweight').

Although most of these tests require sending blood to a pathology laboratory for testing, the development of dry chemistry processes for assessing blood lipids, and portable home devices for measuring blood sugars, now allow rapid and reasonably accurate measurements of cholesterol and some other plasma lipids. The process has become so simple that entrepreneurs have taken to providing quick testing (without any element of standardisation) in venues like shopping centres.

Risk measurements for the overweight

Screening for health risk is useful for the overweight as being overweight is itself a health risk. Some simple measures that might be taken, their cut-off points and what they mean are shown below:

Waist circumference

Because abdominal fat is more dangerous than fat stored elsewhere, waist circumference is a good measure of health risk.

Desirable levels: less than 100 cm for Caucasian men; less than 90 cm for Caucasian women

Asians, Indians and Indigenous Australians should be approximately 10 cm less and Pacific Islanders 10 cm more than these levels.

Blood pressure

This is likely to be increased with increased body fat. There is also a genetic component in cases of very high blood pressure, which requires medication. Mild hypertension can be reduced with weight loss and, in particular, increased physical activity.

Desirable levels: less than 120/80 mmol/L

Cholesterol

Cholesterol is a waxy fat-like substance that can clog arteries. There are genetic influences, and total cholesterol is now considered to be only part of the story.

Desirable levels: less than 5.5 mmol/L
Subfractions include:

LDL or 'bad' cholesterol   Desirable levels: less than 3.0 mmol/L
HDL or 'good' cholesterol   Desirable levels: greater than 1.0 mmol/L

Triglyceride

A combination of potentially dangerous fats, particularly in combination with a high waist circumference and high blood pressure and low HDL.

Desirable levels: less than 3.0 mmol/L

Fasting Plasma Glucose (FPG)

A measure of blood sugars indicating risk of diabetes.

Desirable levels: less than 5.5 mmol/L

HbA1C

A longer-term measure of blood sugars over three to six months; less variable than FPG.

Desirable levels: less than 6 per cent

C-Reactive Protein (CRP)

A relatively new test, which measures the 'stiffness' of arteries and hence possible artery damage. Influenced by weight and reduced with weight loss.

Desirable levels: less than 5.0 mg/L

Thyroid function

Not usually a cause of excess weight, although often blamed as such. May be tested as a check.

Desirable levels: 0.2–4.0 mmol/L

Mass cholesterol-screening programs have now been carried out in Australia and overseas. A large scale screening demonstration program on the north coast of New South Wales was shown to be effective in identifying about a third of the population at risk of heart disease because of high cholesterol (James et al. 1989). The implications of the prevalence of high cholesterol for health promotion have been expounded by McMahon (1990), who suggests from a meta-analysis of epidemiological cholesterol studies that a 10 per cent reduction in cholesterol levels in the Australian population could result in the prevention of 20000 deaths owing to heart disease per year.

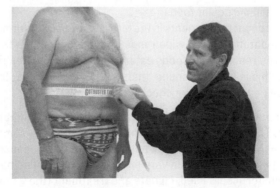

Measuring waist circumference
Fairfax

Dietary assessment

By tradition, dietary assessment has been carried out by qualified dietitians in a clinical setting. The advent of computers and more precise nutrient details (from CSIRO) has meant the development of more reliable computerised nutrition assessment programs.

It is important to remember that nutrition assessments are diagnostic in nature and require interpretation by a qualified professional. Although non-nutritionists could make assessments, any complete program should involve detailed counselling by an appropriate professional. Other means of testing dietary intake are: (a) the diet diary, (b) food recall, and (c) a food intake checklist. The latter can include a check of specific foods eaten such as dietary fat, carbohydrate or drinks, where these are perceived to be a potential problem.

Computerised diet checks—what comes out might not accurately reflect what goes in

Computers have been used in nutrition since the late 1950s, but the advent of personal computers in the 1980s has put computerised diet checks within reach of the ordinary home. A variety of nutrition analysis programs is now commercially available. The difficulty, for someone not versed in nutrition and computers, is how to choose. With prices ranging from a few dollars to several thousand, the wrong choice—for professional or personal use—can be a costly one.

Simplifying computers and diets

In simple terms, computers are a way of counting numbers or estimating quantities. Food is made up of various quantities of chemicals called nutrients. Some of these (e.g. carbohydrate, protein, fats) form a large or important component of most foods, and some (e.g. selenium, manganese) are important in particular foods.

Computers count the nutrients in the total diet by using information stored in a program database for a wide range of commonly eaten foods, and by multiplying the result by the foods eaten over a pre-specified time period.

Although this is logically sound, there are a number of factors that can make or break a computer diet check. For example:

- **The information from which the database is derived might be spurious.** There are many sources of nutrient analysis, some more reliable than others. This should not be unexpected because the nutrient quantity of food can vary enormously depending on where it is grown, fertilisers used, climate and treatment (the vitamin A content of carrots, for example, can vary by 2500 per cent, depending on variety and maturity). Standard nutrient analyses come from recognised government bodies such as the CSIRO or the US Department of Agriculture.

- **The database might not be big enough.** It is difficult to get accurate nutrient analyses for all the thousands of foods that people eat. The size of the database varies from fifty foods to 15000 (obviously the bigger the database, the bigger the computer needed to store it). Usually between 1500 and 1800 items seems to be sufficient and manageable for most purposes.
- **The number of nutrients might be inadequate.** Some databases contain up to seventy nutrients, some of which are of little importance for most purposes. The difficulty is that analyses on many of these nutrients (i.e. certain amino acids) do not exist for many of the foods in the database. Hence, total nutrient analysis can be misleading. The main requirements for general use are the macronutrients (carbohydrates, protein, fat), energy levels (calories or kilojoules), eight to ten vitamins (including A, B1, B2, B3, B6, B12, C, E, pantothenic acid) and three to five minerals (including Ca, An, Fe, Mg).
- **Input might be too complicated.** Input into most programs can be either in numbered codes (representing each food) or as food names. The more modern programs simply require typing the name of the food into the computer, and it is then recognised by the database. Where a food has several subcategories (e.g. corn: fresh cob, tinned, cream), alternatives are posed by the computer and a simple numbered response is required. For those inexperienced with computers, some programs have Help screens so that operations are user-friendly.
- **Output might be inadequate.** Depending on the needs of the user, the output of a diet check program should be informative and educational. At least a printed output of major nutrients and a comparison with recommended daily requirements is required. This should be accompanied by a discussion about each of the critical nutrients in the diet and how the diet could be altered for improvement.
- **Individual differences might not be considered.** The metabolism of foods can vary between individuals and, although it is impossible to predict absorption rates for all nutrients, overall energy usage rates should be able to be measured and taken into consideration in the assessment of energy intake. At present, few diet check programs measure energy output, but those that do are becoming more common.

Fitness and activity assessments

Measuring fitness and activity levels can involve two separate components of measurement. Physical activity is usually measured using a recall or activity check questionnaire. More recently, the advent of pedometers and other movement sensors, which count the number of steps taken over the course of a day, have been used to measure baseline levels of activity as well as prescribe required amounts of activity for health and weight loss benefits.

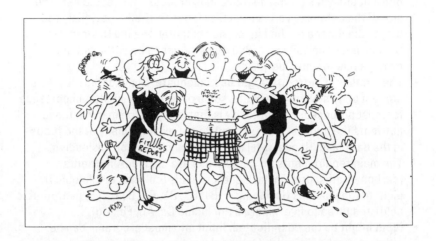

Fitness assessments usually encompass more intrusive measures of physiological capacity. They can consist of a variety of subcomponents, including aerobic fitness, strength, body composition, flexibility, anthropometry and lung capacity. In general, these involve practical measurement techniques that should be performed by qualified exercise personnel (Egger, Champion & Bolton 1998). However, basic fitness testing can be carried out in many cases by trained subprofessional 'fitness leaders' and personal trainers, who might or might not be qualified health promotion practitioners.

Computerised scoring of fitness tests is also available, and it can vary from relatively cheap and simple programs to expensive, detailed, advanced versions. Currently, computerised government fitness testing programs are not widely available, but departments of sport and recreation in most states are able to provide resources and information.

Fitness assessments can be carried out in commercial fitness centres, medical practices, community health centres, the workplace and even the home. Testing is usually used as a basis for developing individualised fitness programs, which again requires the skill of a qualified exercise professional. In some states, testing is now carried out by health insurance organisations.

Stress assessment

Stress assessment questionnaires are widely available, and they vary from the simple and unvalidated 'popular-media' form to the more scientific 'state-and-trait' anxiety scores.

One well-accepted and robust source of stress is changes in life events. The Holmes–Rahe (1967) social adjustment rating scale developed in the 1960s is widely regarded as one indicator of this, although it does have its critics. Proof of high stress levels warrants follow up with the patient in the form of counselling, group therapy or the learning of stress management skills.

Table 3.1: Social readjustment rating scale

Life event	Mean value
1. Death of spouse	100
2. Divorce	73
3. Marital separation from spouse	65
4. Detention in prison or other institution	64
5. Death of a close family member	63
6. Major personal injury or illness	53
7. Marriage	50
8. Being dismissed at work	47
9. Marital reconciliation with spouse	45
10. Retirement from work	45
11. Major change in health or behaviour of family member	44
12. Pregnancy	40
13. Sexual difficulties	39
14. Gaining a new family member (through birth, adoption or an older parent moving in)	39
15. Major business readjustment (merger, reorganisation, bankruptcy)	39
16. Major change in financial state (a lot worse off or a lot better off than usual)	38
17. Death of a close friend	37
18. Changing to a different line of work	36
19. Major change in the number of arguments with spouse (either a lot more or a lot less than usual)	35
20. Taking on a large mortgage (purchasing a home, business)	31
21. Foreclosure on a mortgage or loan	30
22. Major change in responsibilities at work (promotion, demotion, lateral transfer)	29
23. Son or daughter leaving home (marriage, attending school)	29
24. In-law trouble	29
25. Outstanding personal achievement	28
26. Wife beginning or ceasing work outside the home	26
27. Beginning or ceasing formal schooling	26
28. Major change in living conditions (building a new home, remodelling, deterioration of home or neighbourhood)	25
29. Revision of personal habits (dress, manners, associations)	24
30. Troubles with the boss	23

Based on Holmes & Rahe 1967

Individual educational materials

Educational materials for patients and individuals can be in several forms. They can be informational (e.g. pamphlets on health and nutrition), prescriptional (e.g. nutrition for diabetics, exercise for cardiac rehabilitation), contractual (e.g. statement of intent to quit smoking) or evaluational (e.g. progress charts for weight control and stress management).

Much information is already available from various sources. Assessment of existing material should be based on the following questions.

- *Does it appeal to the senses?* Good-quality educational material should be consonant with the aspirations and needs of the reader. It should look attractive and presentable and be easy to understand.
- *Is it culturally specific?* Material promoting the eating of pork is unlikely to be accepted in a large Jewish community, and the promotion of non-indigenous values might have little motivational value to indigenous groups. Where possible, material should be produced within a culture itself and in the language of that culture. Pasick, D'Onofrio and Otero-Sabogal (1996) have suggested that effective health promotion programs will tailor interventions and materials by culture as necessary, but reach across cultures when possible and appropriate. Kreuter and McClure (2004) suggest that culture is particularly relevant when considering the source, the message and channel factors in communications.
- *Is the reading comprehension level appropriate?* It is a common axiom adopted by the popular press that the reading age of the average reader is around the early teens. Although this is not always so, it is true that it is a mistake to make over-optimistic assumptions about comprehension levels, even in professional groups. Of course, the reverse—that is, being patronising—is also a danger.
- *Is the information accurate?* Health professionals and scientists are often pedantic about small matters that they have been involved with for many years. Materials should always be checked for accuracy with specialists in the field to avoid embarrassment once materials are released.
- *Does it achieve its objective?* The objective of any patient educational material needs to be clearly stated. Is it to provide knowledge, change attitudes or influence behaviour? Different objectives will influence both the presentation and the content of materials.

Existing educational resources

A range of patient education materials is available from government departments of health and community services. In addition, a variety of other materials can be readily and cheaply obtained from a variety of sources, such as the following.

- *Australian Society for the Study of Obesity* (ASSO) has downloadable fact sheets on weight control.
- *National Heart Foundation (Australia and New Zealand)* has materials on nutrition, heart disease, exercise.
- *State Cancer Councils* have materials on all forms of cancer, smoking and nutrition.
- *State government departments of sport and recreation* have materials on exercise, recreation and water safety.
- *Australian Nutrition Foundation* has reliable information on nutrition.
- *Private sector*: materials related to products being sold are available. Some might not be seen as impartial (e.g. information on sugar from the sugar industry), but others are prepared in conjunction with impartial bodies, such as the Royal Australian College of General Practitioners.
- *Health insurance organisations*: because they have a vested interest in keeping people well, these organisations are motivated to produce high-quality, useful health information.
- *Medical and pharmaceutical societies*: various medical and pharmaceutical societies and specialty groups (e.g. diabetes, asthma) produce accurate and useful information in the area; medical organisations have become increasingly active in producing health educational material, including videos.

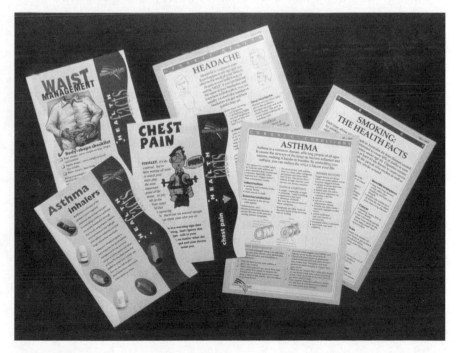

Fact cards from the Pharmacy Self-Care Program

- *Professional associations*: professional organisations—such as the Public Health Association of Australia and New Zealand or the Australian Council for Health, Physical Education and Recreation (ACHPER)— sometimes receive grants to produce materials in their area of expertise.
- *Private organisations*: there are health newsletters such as *Health Yourself* for industry and the *Health Reader* for the professional and interested lay reader; many health videos are now also available on loan from major video-hire outlets.
- *Internet*: the health resources on the Internet are multiplying at an extraordinary rate. Effective categorisation of many of these is available through such documents as WebDoctor (Sharp & Sharp 1998).

Conclusion

Although the economics of health dictate that health promotion practitioners appeal to as wide an audience as possible, certain aspects of health promotion call for an individual focus. Patient education, although individual in orientation, also involves the development of materials with scope for wider usage. Other techniques, such as risk factor screening—although costly and time-consuming—are useful tools for the health promotion practitioner, whether working in the individual, group or whole population setting.

Career opportunities in health promotion

The range of individual approaches to health promotion considered here presents a variety of new and existing career options for health promotion practitioners. Clinical counselling is available through allied health professionals, such as dietitians, psychologists and alternative health practitioners. However, there is a growing need for lifestyle and metabolic counsellors with knowledge in exercise, nutrition and psychology and skills in counselling to work in medical clinics and in shared care with other disciplines. Patient education is available in a number of different areas, including hospitals, community health centres, home care and private consulting. Patient education can also include health professional—or 'train-the-trainer'—options, such as teaching of doctors, nurses, fitness leaders and other health specialists about lifestyle-based health. New opportunities exist in developing Internet sites and programmed learning for specialist areas, such as diabetes, weight control and heart disease, and this could be done with the aid of sponsors or on a fee-for-service basis. Risk factor analysis and health programming are further specialties developed in particular by personal trainers and lifestyle counsellors.

References

Ahrens, R. A., Hower, M., & Best, A. M., 2003, 'Effects of weight reduction interventions by community pharmacists', *J Am Pharm Assoc* 43(5):583–9.

AIHW (Australian Institute of Health and Welfare), 2004, *The Burden of Disease and Injury in Australia*, Canberra, AIHW.

Anderson, P. J., Baade, P. D., Stanton, W. R., & Balanda, K. P., 1995, 'Hospital staff perceptions of health promotion activities in public hospitals', *Health Prom J Aust* 5(3):45–8.

Bessell, T. L., McDonald, S., Silagy, C. A., Anderson, J. N., Hiller, J. E., & Sansom, L. N., 2002, 'Do Internet interventions for consumers cause more harm than good? A systematic review', *Health Expect* 5(1):28–37.

Bonevski, B., Sanson-Fisher, R. W., & Campbell, E., 1996, 'Primary care practitioners and health promotion: a review of current practices', *Health Prom J Aust* 6(1):22–31.

Brankston, G. N., Mitchell, B. F., Ryan, E. A., & Okun, N. B., 2004, 'Resistance exercise decreases the need for insulin in overweight women with gestational diabetes mellitus', *Am J Obstet Gynecol* 190:188–93.

Brett, H., Miller, G. C., Knox, S. et al., 2004, 'General practice activity in the states and territories of Australia 1998–2003', AIHW Cat. No. GEP. 15, Canberra (Australian Institute of Health and Welfare General Practice Series No. 15).

Carmichael, J. M., Alvarez, A., Chaput, R., DiMaggio, J., Magallon, H., & Mambourg, S., 2004, 'Establishment and outcomes of a model primary care pharmacy service system', *Am J Health Syst Pharm* 61(5):472–82.

Celler, B. G., Lovell, N. H., & Basilakis, J., 2003, 'Using information technology to improve the management of chronic disease', *Med J Aust* 179:242–5.

Chandra, A., Malcolm, N., & Fetters, M., 2003, 'Practicing health promotion through pharmacy counseling activities', *Health Prom Pract* 4(1):64–71.

DHSH (Department of Human Services and Health), 1996, Fact Sheets on General Practice, Canberra.

Dijkstra, R. F., Braspenning, J. C., Huijsmans, Z., Peters, S., van Ballegooie, E., ten Have, P., Casparie, A. F., Grol, R. P., 2004, 'Patients and nurses determine variation in adherence to guidelines at Dutch hospitals more than internists or settings', *Diabet Med* 21(6):586–91.

Egger, G., Bolton, A., O'Neill, M., & Freeman, D., 1996, 'Effectiveness of an abdominal obesity reduction program in men: the Gutbuster "waist-loss" programme', *Int J Obes* 20:227–31.

Egger, G., Cameron-Smith, D., & Stanton, R., 2003, *Alternative Treatments for Weight Loss*, Progress in Obesity Research series, John Libbey Eurotext, London.

Egger, G., Champion, C. N., & Bolton, A., 1998, *The Fitness Leader's Handbook* (3rd edn), Kangaroo Press, Sydney.

Egger, G., Fitzgerald, W., Frape, G., Monaem, A., Rubinstein, P., Tyler, C., & Mackay, B., 1983, 'Results of a large-scale media anti-smoking campaign in Australia: the North Coast Healthy Lifestyle Programme', *Brit Med J* 287:1125–87.

Egger, G., & Thorburn, A., 2004, 'Environmental and policy approaches: alternative methods of dealing with obesity', in Kopleson et al. (eds), *Clinical Obesity and Related Metabolic Disorders*, Blackwell Publishing, London.

Falvo, D. R., 2004, *Effective Patient Education: A Guide to Increased Compliance* (3rd edn), Jones & Bartlett, Sudbury, Mass.

Faxman, B., & Eddington, D. W., 1987, 'The accuracy of health-risk appraisal in predicting mortality', *Am J Pub Health* 77(8):971–4.

Gallagher, M., 1989, 'HIV prevention in general practice', *Practitioner* 233:942–3.

General Practice Consultative Committee, 1992, *The Future of General Practice: A Strategy for the Nineties and Beyond*, Australian Medical Association, Parkes, ACT.

Girgis, A., & Sanson-Fisher, R., 1996, 'Community-based health education: general practitioners' perceptions of their role and willingness to participate', *Aust & NZ J Pub Health* 20(4):381–5.

Goode, J. V., Swiger, K., & Bluml, B. M., 2004, 'Regional osteoporosis screening, referral, and monitoring program in community pharmacies: findings from Project ImPACT: Osteoporosis', *J Am Pharm Assoc* 44(2):152–60.

Gruber, W., Llewellyn, J., Arras, C., & Lion, S., 1997, 'The role of the pharmaceutical industry in promoting patient education', *Pat Ed Counsel* 26(1–3):245–9.

Haddock, J., & Burrows, C., 1997, 'The role of the nurse in health promotion: an evaluation of a smoking-cessation programme in surgical pre-admission clinics', *J Advanced Nursing* 26(6):1098–110.

Hickman, M., Drummond, N., & Grimshaw, J., 1994, 'A taxonomy of shared care for chronic disease', *J Public Health Med* 16(4):447–54.

Holmes, T. H., & Rahe, R. H., 1967, 'The Social Readjustment Scale', *J Psychon Res* 11:213–18.

James, R., Tyler, C., Van Beurden, E., & Henrikson, D., 1989, 'Implementing a public cholesterol-screening campaign: the north coast experience', *Commun Health Stud* XIII(2):130–9.

Kirk, A., Mutrie, N., MacIntyre, P., & Fisher, M., 2003, 'Increasing physical activity in people with diabetes', *Diab Care* 26(4):1186–92.

Kreuter, M. W., & McClure, S. M., 2004, 'The role of culture in health communication', *Ann Rev Pub Health* 25:439–55.

Lorig, K., 2000, *Patient Education: A Practical Approach* (3rd edn), Sage Publications, Thousand Oaks, Calif.

Lorig, K. R., & Holman, H., 2003, 'Self-management education: history, definition, outcomes, and mechanisms', *Ann Behav Med* 26(1):1–7.

McMahon, S., 1990, 'Health promotion and cardiovascular risk factors', paper presented to the Public Health Association Health Promotion Division Annual Meeting, Melbourne, Vic.

Meyer, M., 2004, 'Physician use of email: the telephone of the 21st century?', *J Med Pract Manage* 19(5):247–51.

Miles, J., Petrie, C., & Steel, M., 2000, 'Slimming on the Internet', *J R Soc Med* 93(5):254–7.

Osborne, R. H., Spinks, J. M., & Wicks, I. P., 2004, 'Patient education and self-management programs in arthritis', *Med J Aust* 180:S23–6.

Owen, N., 1988, 'Mediated instruction for smoking cessation: hooks, kits and audiovisual materials', in Byrne, D. (ed.), *Smoking Behaviour and its Treatment*, ANU Press, Canberra.

Pasick, R. J., D'Onofrio, C. N., & Otero-Sabogal, R., 1996, 'Similarities and differences across cultures: questions to inform a third generation for health promotion research', *Health Ed Quart* 23 (Suppl 1).S142–61.

Redman, B. K., 2001, *Patient Education* (9th edn), C. V. Mosby, St Louis.

Richards, D., Toop, L., Brockway, K., Graham, S., McSweeney, B., MacLean, D., Sutherland, M., & Parsons, A., 2003, 'Improving the effectiveness of smoking cessation in primary care: lessons learned', *NZ Med J* 116:1173.

Richmond, R. L., Novak, K., Kehoe, L., Calfas, G., & Mendelsohn, C. P., 1998, 'Effect of training on general practitioners' use of a brief intervention for excessive drinkers', *Aust & NZ J Pub Health* 22:206–9.

Roche, A., Bennetts, A., & Mira, M., 1994, 'General practitioners and patient education: attitudes and use of resources', *Health Prom J Aust* 4(2):59–64.

Roland, M., & Dixon, M., 1989, 'Randomised controlled trial of an educational booklet for patients presenting with back pain in general practice', *J Royal Coll Gen Pract* (39):244–6.

Rollnick, S., Heather, N., & Bell, A., 1992, 'Negotiating behaviour change in medical settings: the development of brief motivational interviewing', *J Mental Health* 1:25–37.

Sharp, R. M., & Sharp, V. F., 1998, *Webdoctor: Your Online Guide to Health Care and Wellness*, Quality Medical Publishing Inc., St Louis.

Sherwood, N. E., Morton, N., Jeffery, R. W., French, S. A., Neumark-Sztainer, D., & Falkner, N. H., 1998, 'Consumer preferences in format and type of community-based weight control programs', *Am J Health Promot* 13(1):12–18.

Sinclair, H. K., Bond, C. M., & Stead, L. F., 2004, 'Community pharmacy personnel interventions for smoking cessation', *Cochrane Database Syst Rev* (1):CD003698.

Thomas, R., Cahill, J., & Santilli, L., 1997, 'Using an interactive computer game to increase skill and self-efficacy regarding safer sex negotiation: field test results', *Health Education and Behaviour* 24(1):71–86.

Wallace, P., Cutler, A., & Haines, F., 1988, 'Randomised controlled trial of general practitioner intervention in patients with excessive alcohol consumption', *Brit Med J* 297:663–8.

Watkins, C. J., Papacosta, A. O., Chinn, S., & Martin, J. A., 1987, 'A randomised controlled trial of an information booklet for hypertensive patients in general practice', *J Royal Coll Gen Pract* 7:548–50.

WHO (World Health Organization), 1983, *Primary Health Care in Industrialised Countries: Report on the 1983 Conference in Bordeaux on Primary Health Care in Industrialised Countries*, EURO Reports and Studies, Copenhagen.

—— 1991, *Healthy Hospitals: Next Steps on the Way to the Health-Promoting Hospital*, Budapest Declaration on Health-Promoting Hospitals, WHO, Budapest.

Chapter 4
Focus on groups

Summary of main points

- Groups offer an intermediate approach between one-on-one and population health promotion techniques.
- Health promotion in groups can be either didactic or experiential, and the choice depends on circumstances as well as the intended audience.
- Group skills include an understanding of the processes of learning, group dynamics and communications.
- Most school and higher-level education occurs in groups.
- Group work can include 'train-the-trainer' options and capacity building.
- Advances in interactive technology have expanded the possibilities for group work in health promotion.

If only on grounds of cost-effectiveness, individual strategies in health promotion are usually complemented by strategies that reach a wider audience. Group techniques offer an intermediate approach between one-to-one processes and wider community-focused campaigns. Not only is the group process a key modality for implementing health promotion programs, but also it has been used for many years by other professionals, such as adult education specialists, social workers and psychologists.

Groups can range in size from two or three people to several hundred, and can be homogeneous or heterogeneous in nature. Health promotion methods in such groups are classified here as didactic (i.e. lectures, seminars) or experiential (i.e. skills training, role-playing, simulation/games). This classification is somewhat arbitrary, and others use a range of different classifications (see for example Johnson & Johnson 2002; Corey & Corey 2001; Corey 2003). In line with the rationale of this book, our dichotomy puts the emphasis on process rather than on content, setting or program. The didactic method emphasises, but is not restricted to, persuasion or knowledge transmission ('predisposing' factors), whereas the experiential approach emphasises skills training ('enabling' factors—see Green & Kreuter 1999). A third, but different, use of groups in health promotion is as a source of information. Focus groups for example can be used in formative research (Krueger & Casey 2000; Basch 1987). In contrast to didactic and experiential approaches, which are used primarily to impart information to group participants, focus groups are used to gain information from participants, which can then be used to help structure later health promotion initiatives. Focus groups will be considered in more detail when we discuss social marketing in chapter 5.

The ultimate goal of group methods as used by health promotion practitioners is to empower individuals, organisations and communities by:

- assisting individuals to modify or maintain health-related behaviour
- providing a supportive setting for individuals sharing a common goal or problem
- organising members of a community or an organisation to improve their capacity to identify and solve their own problems (i.e. capacity building or community organisation)
- organising individuals and groups to undertake macro-level social change (e.g. training community leaders, coalition building)
- developing personal health and peer support programs in schools

and, in the case of focus groups, by

- helping health promotion practitioners to plan programs more accurately.

Group methods can be used in a range of different settings, classified by the level of prevention:

- primary prevention: in schools, workplaces and organisations;
- secondary prevention: in medical practices, community health centres, outpatient clinics and drug-referral centres, or
- tertiary prevention: in hospitals, rehabilitation centres and nursing homes.

What is a group?

For health promotion application, Loomis' (1979) definition of a group still applies:

> A group is a collection of individuals who are to some degree interdependent. Within this definition, a number of people waiting for the elevator do not constitute a group. If that same collection of individuals needs to decide whether or not they will allow smoking on the elevator, then they become a group for the purpose of making that decision. Their common task has made them interdependent and therefore a group.

Group behaviour in the influence process has been studied for some time, in parallel with the growth of group psychotherapy processes begun by the early psychoanalysts in the 1920s and 1930s. In the 1960s—an era of unprecedented growth in the study of interpersonal relations and personal awareness—these two lines of development converged. The differences between group processes for the sick and learning practices for the well were broken down, and cross-cultivation of skills emerged. Since that time, groups have become applied to just about every health-related issue from losing weight to learning natural childbirth. (See the box 'Self-help groups available on the Internet' (p. 91) for a list of self-help groups.) Group processes have also become a study in themselves, with many contemporary exponents (see for example Corey & Corey 2001; Cragan 2003; Johnson & Johnson 2002).

Group dynamics

Group dynamics is the study of the nature and development of groups and the inter-relationship of group members with each other and other organisations. Group process skills are relevant in experiential situations, but are less relevant in the didactic (lecturing) situation. Research on group dynamics has described groups in terms of their leadership, membership, goals, norms and interaction of group members (Cragan 2003).

The characteristics of group communication include the following:

- *Group communication occurs in a system.* This implies that there is a connection between all dimensions involved. The dominance of any one dimension (e.g. leadership, membership) can vary in different types of group, but ultimately it is the system that is affected by changes.
- *Group communication dimensions are simultaneously cause and effect.* A message could affect or be affected by components of the group system, depending on other characteristics of the group.
- *Group communication is dynamic.* Changes that occur in groups are continuous, irreversible and unrepeatable, and the group facilitator must be aware of this in using the group process.
- *Group communication is complex.* Any reduction of the group process to simple unidimensional factors will lead to conclusions on behalf of the facilitator that might be counterproductive in the group process. Group processes, unlike the didactic process, are complex and variable.

Group methods

Each of the different approaches to group health promotion listed below calls for different expertise, and no single health promotion practitioner is likely to be expert in all.

The didactic approach, for example, calls for content knowledge, lecturing skills and the ability to answer questions clearly. The experiential approach demands a sensitivity and awareness of group processes. Qualitative research groups require a different set of skills based on questioning, listening and interpreting. Naturally, there is overlap between approaches: lectures and seminars, for example, are usually more effective when there is two-way interaction between presenter and audience. Similarly, experiential learning can benefit from high content knowledge of a group leader.

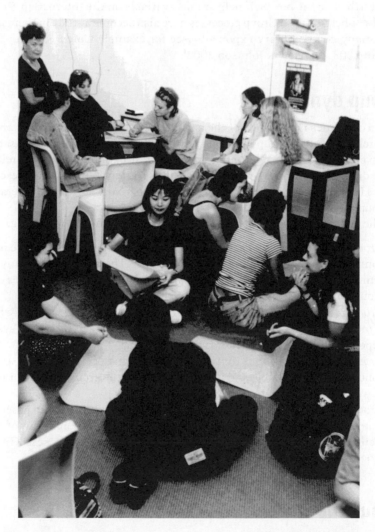

Groups held as part of motivational seminars on nutrition, fitness, self-esteem, drug use and job preparation conducted for young female school leavers by the Smoking and Health Team
Health Department of Western Australia

The didactic method is commonly used when the goal is transmission of knowledge or information. Lectures on HIV/AIDS, for instance, might have as their goal the simple transmission of information about HIV/AIDS risk and risk factor behaviour. As such, the didactic approach is generally individualistic; that is, directed at groups of individuals to bring about individual behaviour change. There are occasions, however, when the didactic method could be used to stimulate actions to influence socioenvironmental changes, which might relate more to the social determinants of health; for example, lectures on the environment and pollution.

Experiential group learning is perhaps best performed when the behavioural outcome required is a complex one and requires detailed development of those components that have been identified in health behaviour theory models as influencing behaviour; that is, intentions, attitudes, barriers and beliefs. The 'predisposing' effect of knowledge, attitudes and beliefs about HIV/AIDS (perceived susceptibility) gained from didactic and other methods can be used to motivate individuals to practise and learn skills ('enabling' factors) in the experiential situation.

Case study 4. 1

Weight control group workshops for doctors

Australia has been one of the first countries in the world to offer post-graduate training in weight control and obesity management to general practitioners. Six-hour workshops that include lectures, practical methods, role-playing, case studies and video presentation began in 1997 in Australia and expanded into six different topic areas. In 2002, GPs who had completed at least three workshops were given the opportunity to convert these (with an extra exam and case studies) into a Post-Graduate Medical Certificate in Weight Control and Obesity Management. By 2004 more than 5000 GPs, or 20 per cent of the total practising GPs in the country, had completed at least one level of the workshop. In 2004, new clinical guidelines for weight control, released by the National Health and Medical Research Council (NH&MRC), were incorporated into the program.

An evaluation of the program with a sample of 400 GPs showed that 91 per cent of them surveyed rated the GP workshops as either 'extremely helpful' or 'helpful'. In an open-ended question, factors regarded as most helpful were: ease of use of the new national physical activity guidelines (38 per cent); use of waist circumference as a clinical screening tool (23 per cent); increased confidence or ability in being proactive in discussing and setting goals (19 per cent), strategies for fat reduction through movement and/or dietary changes (17 per cent); and the importance of weight loss maintenance advice (14 per cent).

Other results were: 69 per cent of GPs claimed to 'definitely' feel more confident and 27 per cent to 'possibly' feel more confident in helping patients with their weight; 45 per cent claimed to have broached the subject of weight loss with patients, even when it might not have been the reason for the consultation (53 per cent claimed they were already doing so); and 48 per cent claimed to have had more weight loss success with patients. In reaction to their increased emphasis on weight management, 31 per cent reported patient responses to this as 'very positive', 60 per cent 'appreciative' and only 4 per cent 'annoyed', 'offended' or 'very negative'.

Importantly, 28 per cent of GPs claimed to have lost weight or waist size themselves, or changed their own habits after the workshop(s). Eighty-three per cent rated the idea of shared care in weight control as either 'excellent' or 'good'.

Egger et al. 2003

Adult learning

The education of adults, as opposed to children and adolescents, is a multi-faceted, complex process that encompasses many subject and interest areas. A whole area of study has been devoted to the topic since the 1970s (see for example Verduin, Miller & Greer 1979). Because adults have lived for and experienced a given number of years, they have had the opportunity to gain many perceptions of their environment and the objects and events in it. An adult's past experience then forms the basis from which education and behaviour change must commence. Adult behaviour at this stage could be more rigid than that of younger people because adult behaviour has been formed over a longer period of time.

A significant factor in adult learning is the notion of perceived threat. Threat is the perception of an imposed force requiring a change in behaviour, values or beliefs to avert the threat. However, a threat might result in defensive behaviour and a narrowing and constricting of the perceptual field.

Since the modification of perception and behaviour in adult groups is personal and requires attention to threat processing, any adult learning program should be as individual as possible. This requires keeping the individual moving towards their goal. Since retention might be a problem in adult learning situations, it is important to emphasise progress and to reinforce learned practices continually.

Lack of progress in achieving goals among some adult learners can be attributed to low self-esteem and a lack of self-confidence. Account needs to be taken of this, as well as the fact that learning rates might vary among individuals, in the provision of feedback and reward in order to maintain and enhance motivation.

Finally, since adult learning could be a more gradual process than child learning, adults must be given appropriate time and guidance to experience and develop new behaviour. Furthermore, some tasks might take more time to learn and others less, which illustrates again the importance of individual attention. For further information on adult learning principles, see Merriam and Caffarello (1998), Knowles et al. (1998) and Tennant (1997). Other authors (e.g. Corey & Corey 2001) also discuss specific group processes for children, adolescents and the elderly.

Table 4.1 is a summary of the methods and characteristics of group processes. The discussion that follows explains the processes in detail and illustrates the situations in which each might best be utilised.

Table 4.1: A summary of group methods in health promotion

Didactic group methods	Description
Lecture–discussion	Best for knowledge transmission or motivation in large groups. Requires a dynamic, effective speaker with more knowledge than the audience.
Seminar	Smaller numbers (2–20). Leader–group feedback. Leader most knowledgeable in the group. Best for trainer learning.
Conference	Can combine lecture or seminar techniques. Best for professional development.
Video conferencing	Opportunity for group learning with professionals, such as rural and remote doctors, nurses and so on.

Experiential group methods	Description
Skills training	Requires motivated individuals. Includes explanation, demonstration and practice; for example, relaxation, childbirth, exercise.
Behaviour modification	Learning and unlearning of specific habits. Stimulus–response learning. Generally behaviour-specific; for example, smoking cessation, phobia desensitisation.
Inquiry learning	Used mainly in school settings. Requires formulating and problem solving through group cooperation.
Peer group discussion	Useful where shared experiences, support and awareness are important. Participants homogeneous in at least one factor; for example, old people, prisoners, teenagers.
Simulation	Useful for influencing attitudes in individuals with varying abilities. Generally in school setting, but relevant to other groups.
Role-play	Acting of roles by group participants. Can be useful where communication difficulties exist between individuals in a setting; for example families, professional practice. Requires skilled facilitator.
Self-help	Requires motivation and independent attitude. Valuable for ongoing peer support and values clarification. Can be therapy or a forum for social action.

Detailed explanation of methods

Didactic methods

Didactic approaches involve the health promotion practitioner in a predominantly authoritative role with an audience or individual. There are a number of different ways of doing this: lecture or discussion, seminar or workshop, and conference, all of which are discussed below.

Lecture and discussion

The lecture, presentation or talk is one of the oldest teaching methods. Recourse to any historical science book will relate numerous circumstances of seminal lectures—the date, time, place and topic—delivered by now-revered thinkers, which have played a role in changing the face of the world.[1] As a health education practice, however, the lecture–discussion is one of the most difficult to master. Part of the professional process of health promotion practitioners is to be aware of their skills and limitations. If a lecture situation is required, a practitioner who does not have the necessary skills should attempt to develop them, or facilitate other professionals with the appropriate skills. Groups such as Toastmasters and other organisations and associations can help develop these skills.

The advantages of the lecture are that it is easy to use, can impart information, can influence opinion, and can stimulate thought and critical thinking. Lectures are economical and practical, and can incorporate dialogue between the lecturer and participants. The disadvantages are that lecturing involves skills that might be difficult for the lecturer to master, that the audience is generally passive (and therefore less likely to learn in some cases), and that the lecture approach is not suited to the learning of complex skills.

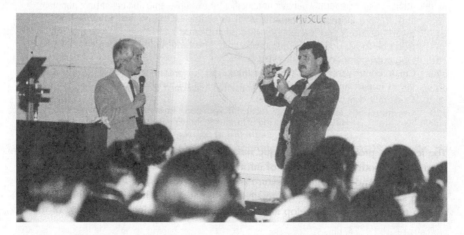

The lecture style is a longstanding method of health promotion

The efficacy of the lecture as a means of education is unquestioned. What is less certain, however, is the comparative effectiveness of the lecture in contrast to other techniques (discussion groups, educational films, video). Indeed, each technique has its advantages in different conditions. Research carried out by Green (1978) found that the lecture is less effective than group discussion and other methods where there is a need for attitudinal change or the development of problem-solving or values-clarification skills. It is also probable that the didactic approach works differently for different audiences. Case study 4.1 discussed use of the lecture approach with doctors, who, because of their objective training in physiological information and their cognitive ability, respond well to this approach.

The lecture is probably the technique most used by health educators and other health practitioners, both for the transmission of information to the public and for the training of professional groups. Although the lecture is a valuable technique, it can be overused and used in situations where it is not appropriate. The challenge for the health promotion practitioner is to develop an educational mix, which includes the use of the lecture in appropriate situations.

Tips for planning a good lecture

1. Know your subject, or at least that part of it you are going to speak about.
2. Prepare audiovisuals to accompany your main points.
3. Speak slowly and clearly, and use a microphone if there are more than a few people.
4. Make eye contact with the audience.
5. Always look at the audience; don't talk to the screen.
6. Plan your timing closely and avoid the number 1 sin: going over time.
7. Don't go too slowly at the start and then have to speed up to get the main points in.
8. Tell them what you're going to tell them; tell them; then tell them what you told them.
9. Never admit to the audience that you are nervous or scared!
10. Remember, it takes a lifetime for someone to find out what you know, but only one sentence to find out what you don't!

If using a PowerPoint presentation:

- Present issues one at a time.
- Make the best use of colour.
- Make use of contrast in colours.
- Don't put too much on one screen.
- Consider short videos embedded in the presentation if they make a point.
- Use fewer overheads rather than too many.
- Use PowerPoint as an adjunct to your presentation, not as the presentation itself.

The lecture–discussion method is appropriate when:

- information transmission and motivation are the main goals
- the lecturer knows more than the group about the subject
- the group is too large for small group activity
- all participants need to hear the same information in the same way
- the lecturer is a dynamic, informative and sensitive speaker, and
- the audience is reasonably motivated, aware of and interested in the topic.

Seminar/workshop

The seminar involves elements of the lecture–discussion approach with more group interaction. Generally, the numbers involved are smaller (between two and fifteen), allowing greater interaction with the seminar leader.

The main difference between the seminar and the experiential technique is that seminars are generally more information-based rather than skills-based, and involve some didactic discussion from a leader with greater knowledge of content than the group. Seminars are most effective in training of trainers or other health professionals, when it is important for the leader to get feedback about learning from the group. The seminar method is most appropriate when:

- small numbers are involved
- feedback to the lecturer from participants is important
- groups are homogeneous (e.g. diabetics, asthmatics, nurses)
- there are limitations of space and time
- professional training is required, and
- the seminar leader knows more about the topic than the group.

Conference

A conference is usually a combination of the lecture and seminar/workshop techniques. It is usually reserved for professional development and networking and is generally conducted over several hours or days. The conference usually requires several 'keynote' authorities in the subject areas, and can be conducted with large groups of people (in large and smaller groups). Conference delegates usually get their own opportunity to present information or research via proffered papers, often to smaller audiences, depending on the number of conference attendees. Conferences are generally about a specific topic or subject area. The conference method is appropriate when:

- professional updating of information is required
- several experts in the field can be involved
- there is a need for consensus among professionals, and
- participants have basic knowledge in the area.

Suitability for the didactic approach

Appropriate subjects for the didactic approach include lectures on:

- HIV/AIDS
- lifestyle
- risk factors
- parenthood
- baby health
- nutrition
- exercise, and
- immunisation.

Less appropriate situations for the didactic approach include:

- community development
- stress management
- quit-smoking training
- drug therapy
- mental health
- family therapy
- weight control, and
- peer support.

Case study 4.2

Preventing scalds in New Zealand school children

A scalds prevention program for school groups involving just two classroom sessions and a homework exercise that targeted five safety practices shows the value of this type of education in the long term. The program was taught to twenty-eight classes in fourteen schools in Waitakere City, New Zealand, by public health nurses (PHNs). Children aged 10–11 from three of the schools in ethnically diverse, low- to middle-income areas were then assessed for their knowledge of scalds hazards a year after the program. They recalled a mean of 7.46 out of 10 hazards. Altogether, 65–79 per cent of children reported that each of the five safety practices provided were at least temporarily used as intended, and 29–55 per cent reported that they were still in use a year later. Interviews with children's parents indicated that the majority of their hot water practices had not been optimally safe before the program and that many had adopted the suggested practices. While the PHNs were positive about the program, they suggested teachers could also deliver it as part of the school curriculum.

Moore, Morath & Harre 2004

Experiential methods

'I hear and I forget. I see and I remember. I do and I understand.'

Confucius

Working with small groups

Working with groups is a key role of the health promotion practitioner, whether it be focus groups (in needs assessment and planning), discussion groups (for education and awareness-raising), or learning groups (for behaviour modification skills training).

In some respects small groups, as used in health promotion, are similar to processes involved in focus group interviews. The focus group interview is a qualitative research technique used to obtain data about perceptions, feelings and opinions of small groups of participants about a given problem, experience, service, product or other phenomenon (for more on focus groups in social marketing see chapter 5). Focus group research is concerned with eliciting and understanding concepts rather than with measuring them; for example expanding knowledge, identifying and clarifying issues, identifying behaviour, explaining behaviour, generating hypotheses and providing input into future research.

Characteristics of small groups as used in health promotion are:

- the size of the group is usually six to twelve participants (although this is flexible, and productive sessions can be conducted with fewer or more participants)
- discussions usually last one to three hours
- a 'safe' or non-threatening setting (physically and psychologically) is required
- the group leader or facilitator requires skill in facilitating effective communication and is of key importance to the success of the outcome, and
- concerns, experiences and motives might be the subject of discussions.

Tactics of the group facilitator

Interpersonal tactics useful in the group situation include the following:

- *Be non-judgmental.* If group members feel that their opinions, attitudes and behaviour are likely to be judged as good or bad by the facilitator, they are less likely to contribute openly. This does not always mean agreeing with the attitudes and behaviour of others, but it does mean acceptance of differences.
- *Be honest.* Sharing thoughts and feelings with a group is important in developing an open and trusting atmosphere. A willingness to do so by the facilitator can be a catalyst for others to contribute.

- *Foster trust*. This is an ongoing development that depends on the feedback that the group members receive from each other and the facilitator. If they feel accepted as worthwhile members of the group, trust in the group will develop.
- *Observe*. The facilitator needs to be a sensitive observer of the interactions, behaviour and underlying processes occurring in the group. If direction is lost, or the task becomes confused, it is up to the facilitator to get the group back on track with as little disruption as possible.
- *Be sensitive*. Group members might sometimes share personal experiences that are personal and important to them. The facilitator needs to be sensitive to individuals' needs in order to aid the total group process.
- *Communicate*. Effective communication is both verbal and non-verbal. In some situations (e.g. focus groups), it is important for facilitators to stay quiet so that their ideas do not influence the needs-assessment process. However, non-verbal cues—such as head nodding and shrugging could be just as potent. Communication means not just listening to words but also tuning in to the other person's feelings. Effective communication by the facilitator will establish the opportunity for all to contribute and to feel valued as group members.
- *Be flexible*. Leadership styles vary according to the nature of a group and the stage of the group's development. For example, early in a group's life, more structure and direction could be required. As the group develops, the tasks might be developed and relationships in the group maintained with little direction from the facilitator.
- *Be firm*. It is inevitable that occasions will arise when group members display behaviour that might be disruptive to the group. Aggression, dominance of the discussions and other disruptive behaviour can cause others to become defensive, withdrawn or frustrated by the group's interaction. If left unchecked by the facilitator, such behaviour can result in a dysfunctional group.

Skills training

This involves the group learning of skills that can facilitate the health process; that is, stress management, healthy cooking, prenatal breathing, self-care and so on. The skill development method should provide explanation about the need for a procedure, demonstration of the procedure for the group and practical experience in the procedure.

Skills development can include training in communication for conflict resolution, self-assertion and group decision making. The procedure has been used in school health education programs to teach adolescents how to cope with peer pressure to smoke or take drugs (Botvin, Eng & Williams 1980). Computer programs have been developed to assist young people in the development of life skills. For example, SMART Talk—a multimedia, computer-based, violence prevention intervention—employs games, simulations, graphics, cartoons and interactive interviews to engage young adolescents in learning new skills to resolve conflicts without violence (Bosworth et al. 1996).

Skills training is most effective when techniques are required for 'coping' with situations that might be adverse to health. It should be used only with participants whose values and intentions have been clearly defined.

Health promotion practitioners utilising small group methods frequently in their roles could benefit from formal training in group facilitation techniques available from reputable training organisations in most capital cities and some regional centres. Certain group topics—such as stress management, inter-personal communication skills training, role-play and exercise instruction—are a useful addition to any health promoter's armoury. These can be learned from a number of sources (e.g. Lawson & Callaghan 1991; Johnson & Johnson 2002). For other, more specific skills training, the practitioner can draw on specialist expertise such as that of counsellors and psychologists.

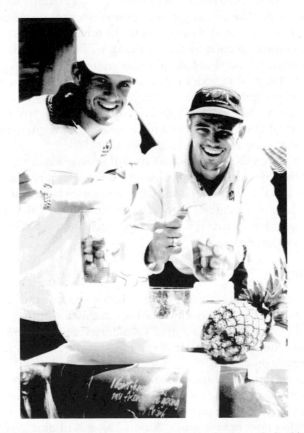

Professional footballers doing taste testing at a stall teaching how to make healthy 'mocktails'
Health Department of Western Australia

Behaviour modification

Behaviour modification is the specific process of learning and unlearning habits based on stimulus–response learning theory. The process requires the facilitator to have skills, knowledge and an understanding of learning theory principles, such as reinforcement (anything that increases a response), punishment (anything that decreases a response), stimulus generalisation (responding to cues that are similar to the originally conditioned cue), and extinction (when a response ceases because it is no longer reinforced).

Behaviour modification can be carried out in groups or individually and is generally used to unlearn unhealthy habits, although the method can be used to develop healthy habits as a component of other health promotion programs, such as exercise. Behaviour modification is most suited to situations that involve individuals who are motivated and informed but have difficulty breaking old habits (Norman, Abraham & Connor 2000). Examples include quit smoking, weight control, diet and anxiety reduction programs.

Inquiry learning

Inquiry learning has developed under the patronage of psychologist Jerome Bruner (1966). In this process, often used in schools, group participants are encouraged to formulate and test their own hypotheses, which they can do in small groups, through practical excursions, reading and personal experience.

The inquiry learning approach is applicable to some community group settings—for example patient–doctor interactions—although it is not often used by health promotion practitioners.

Case study 4.3

School groups, soft drink consumption and health promotion practice

As with any new claim against vested interests in health, the first stage is often one of denial or the claim that there is 'no convincing evidence' of a connection between a manufacturer's product and ill-health. Reaction from the tobacco industry against claims initially made in 1950 continued in this fashion for three to four decades, despite more than 50 000 research articles proving a link between smoking and cancer. More recently, a link between soft drink consumption and obesity was found by British researchers who found a reduction in soft drink use and weight losses in children from schools where group education about the risks of soft drink use was carried out, compared to control schools where this did not occur. This is likely to increase demands on soft drink control as a public health measure.

James et al. 2004

Peer group discussion/support

Discussion methods are often regarded as superior to the lecture method when a homogeneous group with a common purpose exists. In the schools situation, this is often practised to develop an understanding and awareness of the processes of peer pressure involved in many health-associated forms of behaviour (e.g. drinking, drug-taking, sexual activity). Peer groups are useful for shared experiences, group support, awareness raising and idea generation. Peer education programs have also been employed successfully in the delivery of health education programs for HIV/AIDS among high-risk populations (Dark 1996). With a skilful leader, groups such as senior citizens, prisoners, patients and students can benefit from the peer group discussion–interaction process. The technique also involves processes included in other group methods (i.e. sensitivity groups and role-play).

The introduction of the Internet and chat rooms has made the discussion method a popular one for widespread group involvement with people who have something in common. No doubt many more opportunities will develop in this area as the technology expands.

Simulation

'Simulation' refers to the process of enacting a real-life experience. Simulation learning in groups can take the form of games, dramatisation, role-play, case studies and repeats of actual experience. Where simulations are carried out, group leaders should be well prepared, know the outcome of the process and be ready for appropriate actions and questions.

Because of their nature as games, simulations have usually been confined to the school experience. However, there is scope for further development into lifestyle groups and patient education. Simulation appears to be most effective in increasing motivation and influencing attitudes in groups with a wide range of abilities.

Role-play

Role-play involves acting out an experience in the way an individual would enact that experience. For example, it might involve teenagers in a group talking like the smoker of a particular advertised brand of cigarettes, or adults acting the problems of a drug user in order to understand the problems of that individual.

Role-play can be structured (pre-planned, rehearsed) or unstructured (impromptu). There are five techniques that help the role-play situation:

- *role reversal*: where individuals mimic each other
- *soliloquy*: where the actors are asked about their feelings
- *doubling*: where observers interject their feelings
- *multiple role-playing*: where several participants act each role, and
- *role rotation*: where roles are changed during the action.

Role-playing is most useful in schools, in situations where people have difficulty expressing their thoughts about each other (i.e. in family education) and where roles are a significant hindrance to the health process (van Ments 1989), for example where being an 'alpha male' means not accepting the need to check health risks.

Self-help groups

Self-help has been discussed as an individual process in chapter 3. Self-help groups now also exist in a range of different health-related areas (e.g. alcohol and drug abuse, domestic violence, weight control, gambling, parenthood, child abuse, and infectious and chronic diseases), both geographically and through the Internet. Often these carry the epithet '– anonymous' (e.g. Alcoholics Anonymous, Gamblers Anonymous, Over-Eaters Anonymous) to encourage greater participation among those concerned about revealing their identity. The role of the health promotion practitioner is to facilitate and selectively recommend such groups, rather than become involved in the group process as such, which would defeat the main purpose of the group; that is, to develop self-esteem through individual and group action. Self-help groups can have therapy as their main purpose (e.g. drug abuse) or can be community and action-oriented (e.g. Neighbourhood Watch).

Self-help groups available on the Internet

The rise of the Internet has led to a huge increase in the number of self-help groups with immediate access to information on their ailment or condition. In many cases of obscure diseases, this has made patients greater experts than their doctors, and challenges the one-way education process from patient to doctor. Some relevant self-help group sites for prevalent modern disease categories include the following:

- arthritis: www.health.gov.au/pq/arthritis
- asthma: www.asthma.org.au
- depression: www.beyondblue.com.au
- diabetes: www.diabetesincontrol.com
- heartburn (reflux): www.nevdgp.org.au/geninf/gastro/heartbur.htm
- pregnancy: www.med.monash.edu.au/healthpromotion/pamphlets/pregnancy
- sleep apnoea: www.sleepaus.on.net/links.html
- weight control: www.asso.org.au.

General self-help advice or support groups can be found at www.healthinsite. gov.au (Australian Government) and www.drsref.com.au/support.html (Doctor's Reference site).

This list is non-exhaustive and will change over time. Readers are advised to use an Internet search engine to seek out contemporary groups.

Processes are being developed to enable the practitioner to screen individuals for their potential success in self-help therapy groups, and computer programs might assist this process in the future.

Suitability for experiential approach

Appropriate situations for the experiential approach include:

- behaviour learning
- risk factor modification
- interpersonal skills
- substance abuse
- self-care
- quit smoking exercises
- weight control
- family education
- sex education
- coping skills training
- personal hygiene
- family planning, and
- healthy-cooking classes.

Less appropriate situations for the experiential approach include:

- infectious disease information, and
- immunisation education.

Some practicalities

Most people wishing to develop group-learning activities assume that an army of paid group leaders on substantial salaries is a basic requirement. Such an approach is obviously economically impractical. There are, however, effective alternatives using the principles that have been developed in marketing. The essential features are:

- the participants pay
- the income is used to employ group leaders, and
- group leaders are recruited from successful former group participants, who then receive formal training in group facilitation.

Allowances can be made for free participation by low-income earners.

There are many successful examples of this approach with literally thousands of participants from both rich and poor neighbourhoods creating and running groups on topics such as child rearing, stress reduction and weight control. A highly successful example of this technique, which has become a commercial venture, is Weight Watchers International (see case study 4.4).

Case study 4.4

Weight loss in groups: the Weight Watchers model

Weight Watchers was started in the 1960s initially for women to provide group support for fellow women faced with the onerous (and lonely) task of losing weight. The Weight Watchers approach has served as a model for weight control programs ever since. In the process, Weight Watchers has become a multinational organisation with shares on international stock markets. Despite several attempts to broaden the concept to include males, however, its client base remains largely female, probably because of the nature of the group support provided, which has more appeal to women. Although Weight Watchers is commercially sensitive about its results, like most commercial weight loss programs, its limited published data suggests that the program is more effective than self-help in achieving and maintaining weight loss in women.

Heshka et al. 2000

Summary of group methods

The focus on groups in this chapter has concentrated on practical skills useful in modifying health behaviour in a cost-effective manner. These techniques can satisfy the needs of dealing with high-risk individuals in the community but, in general, are likely to have little impact on the structural causes of ill-health.

The population level approaches discussed in the next chapter extend the practitioner's ability to modify the health of individuals in a community, and introduce skills that also act on the social determinants of ill-health.

Career opportunities in health promotion

Career opportunities for health promotion professionals utilising group skills include teaching physical education and/or personal development in schools, or as a fitness or recreation officer in fitness and leisure centres, industry or the armed services. Lecturing, either as a public or motivational speaker, or in an academic capacity, is another option. Opportunities also exist to work as a group moderator or facilitator, for example as a diabetes, arthritis or asthma educator, either privately or for group medical or other practices. Group leaders are often employed by private organisations, such as adventure or personal development organisations or corporate health and fitness programs. Audiovisual production for specific group-based programs is another opportunity, given the increasing need to develop online programs, for example for rural and remote health professionals. This can also include health professional, or 'train-the-trainer', options, such as teaching doctors, nurses, fitness leaders and other health specialists in lifestyle-based health, either face-to-face or in groups.

Note

1 An excellent recent discussion of many of these is contained in Bill
Bryson's popular book, *A Short History of Nearly Everything*, Doubleday,
New York, 2003.

References

Basch, C. E., 1987, 'Focus group interview: an underutilized research
technique for improving theory and practice in health education', *Health
Ed Quart* 14(4):411–48.

Bosworth, K., Espelage, D., DuBay, T., Dahlberg, L. L., & Daytner, G.,
1996, 'Using multimedia to teach conflict-resolution skills to young
adolescents', *Am J Prev Med* 12(Suppl. 5):65–74.

Botvin, G., Eng, A., & Williams, C., 1980, 'Preventing onset of cigarette
smoking through life-skills training', *Prev Med* (9):135–43.

Bruner, J. S., 1966, *Toward a Theory of Instruction*, Harvard University
Press, Cambridge, Mass.

Corey, G., 2003, *Group Techniques* (3rd edn), Brooks/Cole, New York.

Corey, M., & Corey, G., 2001, *Groups: Process and Practice* (6th edn),
Brooks/Cole, New York.

Cragan, J. F., 2003, *Communication in Small Groups: Theory, Process and
Skills* (6th edn), Wadsworth Publishing, Belmont, Calif.

Dark, L. S., 1996, 'Peer approaches for increasing HIV awareness on a college
campus', *ABNF Journal* 7(2):54–6.

Egger, G., & Thorburn, A., 2004, 'Environmental and policy approaches:
alternative methods in dealing with obesity', Kopelson et al. (Eds),
Clinical obesity and related metabolic disorders, Blackwell Publishing,
London.

Green, L. W., 1978, 'Determining the impact and effectiveness of health
education as it relates to federal policy', *Health Ed Monographs* 6(1):28–
66.

Green, L. W., & Kreuter, M. W., 1999, *Health Promotion Planning: An
Educational and Environmental Approach*, Mayfield Publishing Co.,
Mountain View, Calif.

Heshka, S., Greenway, F., Anderson, J. W., Atkinson, R. L., Hill, J. O.,
Phinney, S. D., Miller-Kovach, K., & Xavier Pi-Sunyer, F., 2000, 'Self-help
weight loss versus a structured commercial program after 26 weeks: a
randomized controlled study', *Am J Med* 109(4):282–7.

James, J., Thomas, P., Cavan, D., & Kerr, D., 2004, 'Preventing childhood
obesity by reducing consumption of carbonated drinks: cluster
randomized controlled trial', *Brit J Med* 328:1237–9.

Johnson, D. W., & Johnson, F. P., 2002, *Joining Together: Group Theory and
Group Skills* (8th edn), Prentice Hall, Englewood Cliffs, NJ.

Knowles, M. S., Holton, E. T., & Swanson, R. A., 1998, *The Adult Learner: The Definitive Classic in Adult Education and Human Resource Development* (5th edn), Gulf Publishing, Houston, Tex.

Krueger, R. A., & Casey, M. A., 2000, *Focus Groups: A Practical Guide for Applied Research* (3rd edn), Sage Publications, Thousand Oaks, Calif.

Lawson, J., & Callaghan, A., 1991, 'Recreating the village: focus groups for new mothers', *Aust J Pub Health* 15(1):64–6.

Loomis, M. E., 1979, *Group Processes for Nurses*, C. V. Moseby, St Louis.

Merriam, S. B., & Caffarello, R. S., 1998, *Learning in Adulthood: A Comprehensive Guide* (2nd edn), Jossey-Bass, New York.

Moore, J., Morath, K., & Harre, N., 2004, 'Follow-up study of a school-based scalds prevention programme', *Health Educ Res* May 20.

Norman, P., Abraham, C., & Connor, M., 2000, *Understanding and Changing Health Behaviour: From Health Beliefs to Self-Regulation*, Routledge, New York.

Tennant, M., 1997, *Psychology and Adult Learning*, Routledge, New York.

Van Ments, M., 1989, *The Effective Use of Role Play: A Handbook for Teachers*, Nichols Publishing, New York.

Verduin, J. R., Miller, H. G., & Greer, C. E., 1979, *Adults Teaching Adults*, Learning Concepts, Houston, Tex.

Chapter 5
Focus on populations I:
social marketing and the media

Summary of main points

- Social marketing is the application of commercial marketing techniques to the achievement of socially desirable goals.
- Social marketing is distinguished by a consumer orientation, and hence relies on research to identify, understand, reach and motivate the target audience.
- The media—in all forms—is a crucial component of social marketing and health promotion campaigns, given that our major 'product' is information.
- There are five major media methods: advertising, publicity, edutainment, civic journalism and new interactive technologies, and three major campaign objectives: informing, persuading and advocating.

Health promotion and communities

> A community is a specific group of people usually living in a defined geographical area who share a common culture, are arranged in a social structure, and exhibit some awareness of their identity as a group. In modern societies, individuals rarely belong to a single, distinct 'community' but maintain membership of a range of communities based on variables such as geography, occupation, social contact and leisure interests. (Nutbeam 1986)

According to this definition of community, those health promotion strategies oriented to individuals and groups covered to this point could also be relevant for community programs. In the case of organisational action, for example, the desired outcome might be an influence on a whole community or population group. Community development processes also begin with groups of individuals, although their prime concern is a wider community base. In the case of community-focused health promotion activities, the emphasis is taken off high-risk individuals and placed on lowering the average risk of all individuals in the community.

Influencing community behaviour

At the heart of community interventions is an understanding of the processes of social behaviour. Much has been written on the subject, and many theoretical approaches have been developed. Some accentuate the importance of interpersonal interactions in influencing societal norms and values, which in turn play a key role in shaping societies. Others stress the importance of the individual and the role of personal interest in shaping social actions.

Change can be brought about at the community level, according to Ross and Mico (1980), through all or any of seven different methods, which they list in order from low-resistance to high-resistance modes:

1. *diffusion and adoption*—based on communication and opinion leadership
2. *consensus organising*—coming from shared interests
3. *social planning*—involving citizen participation
4. *political action*—including legislation, lobbying, campaigning
5. *confrontive negotiation*—i.e. threat of reactive action
6. *non-violent disruption*—such as strikes, boycotts, protests
7. *violent disruption*—revolution, riots and so on.

The first of these involves social marketing and mass media. The remainder are more appropriate for community development or organisation, and will be covered in chapter 6.

Social marketing

According to Schwartz (1995), social marketing is a program planning process that promotes voluntary behaviour change on the basis of:

* offering benefits people want
* reducing barriers people face, and
* using persuasion, not just information.

The term 'social marketing' appears to have been used first by Kotler and Zaltman in 1971 to describe the application of the principles and methods of marketing to the achievement of socially desirable goals. Since then, the use of marketing techniques in the health area has grown rapidly in Australia and other industrialised nations as well as in developing countries. The 1980s saw a massive growth both in Australia and overseas, in mass media-based health promotion campaigns utilising marketing concepts, across a broad range of activities, including injury prevention, drinking and driving, seat belt usage, drugs, smoking, exercise, immunisation, nutrition and heart disease prevention (Egger, Donovan & Spark 1993; Fine 1990; Kotler & Roberto 1989; Manoff 1985; Walsh et al. 1993).

A number of factors influenced this trend. One was the realisation by social scientists and health professionals that, although they were expert in assessing what people should do, they were not necessarily expert in communicating these messages, or in motivating or facilitating behavioural change. Another

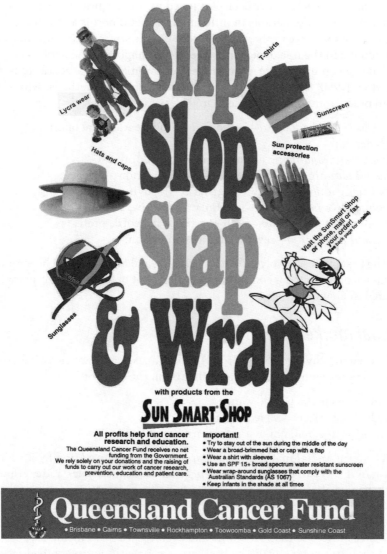

One of Australia's best-known health slogans
Queensland Cancer Fund

influence was the apparent success of marketing techniques in the commercial area and the observation that the discipline of marketing provides a systematic, research-based approach for the planning and implementation of mass intervention programs.

Yet another influence was the move in public health towards the prevention of the so-called lifestyle diseases, such as heart disease and cancer—an approach based on epidemiological research findings about the relationships between habitual behaviour and long-term health outcomes. This focus on lifestyle diseases in turn led to an emphasis (some would say an undue emphasis) on individual responsibility and behaviour change. Hence, there was an increased acceptance of the marketing philosophy of individualism and rational free choice.

Some critics of social marketing have claimed that such a philosophy largely ignores the social, economic and environmental factors that influence individual health behaviour. Some social marketing campaigns deserve this criticism. However, it shows a lack of understanding of social marketing on both sides since one of the fundamental aspects of marketing—and hence social marketing—is an awareness of the total environment in which the organisation operates and how this environment influences, or can itself be influenced, to enhance the marketing activities of the company or health agency (see Donovan & Henley 2003; Hastings & Haywood 1994; Buchanan, Reddy & Hossain, 1994).

The increasing use of marketing practices by non-profit organisations and for social change objectives has in fact led to a redefinition of the term 'marketing' from that used by the American Marketing Association in 1960; that is, 'the performance of business activities that direct the flow of goods and services from producer to consumer or user', to include the marketing of ideas; that is, 'the process of planning and executing the conception, pricing, promotion, and distribution of ideas, goods, and services to create exchanges that satisfy individual and organisational objectives' (*Marketing News* 1985).

Social marketing defined

As first defined by Kotler and Zaltman (1971), social marketing is 'the design, implementation and control of programs calculated to influence the acceptability of social ideas and involving considerations of product planning, pricing, communications and market research'. An often-cited and more recent definition is that of Andreasen (1995): 'Social marketing is the application of commercial marketing technologies to the analysis, planning, execution, and evaluation of programs designed to influence the voluntary behaviour of target audiences in order to improve their personal welfare and that of their society.'

Donovan and Henley (2003) consider Andreasen's definition too constrictive in its emphasis on voluntary behaviour. For example they point out that a social marketing campaign for the National Heart Foundation, with an end goal of individuals consuming less saturated fats, might also target biscuit manufacturers to persuade them to substitute saturated fats in their products with polyunsaturated fats. Whereas this requires a voluntary behaviour change among food company executives, the end-consumers' change in saturated fats intake is involuntary. Hence Donovan and Henley modify Andreasen's definition to 'the application of commercial marketing technologies to the analysis, planning, execution and evaluation of programs designed to influence the voluntary or involuntary behaviour of target audiences in order to improve the welfare of individuals and society'. They add two key points to their approach to social marketing:

- given debate about who decides what is 'good' in the above definitions, they propose the UN Universal Declaration of Human Rights (www. unhchr.ch) as the baseline with respect to the common good, and
- although most social marketing in the public health and injury prevention areas has focused on achieving individual behaviour change, largely independent of the individual's social and economic circumstances, a primary future goal of social marketing is to achieve changes in these social determinants of health and wellbeing.

Hence, under this definition, which is also shared by other writers (e.g. Hastings, McFadyen & Anderson 2000), social marketing is not just the targeting of individual voluntary behaviour change and changes to the environment that facilitate such changes but also the targeting of changes in social structures that will facilitate individuals reaching their potential. This includes the targeting of individuals in communities who have the power to make institutional policy and legislative change.

Social marketing uses key concepts from mainstream product and service marketing: market segmentation; market research; competitive assessment; the use of product, price, promotion and distribution tactics; pre-testing and ongoing evaluation of campaign strategies; and models of consumer behaviour adapted from the psychological and communications literature.

For many health promotion professionals, social marketing is seen as synonymous with the use of mass media to promote socially desirable causes. This view is not unexpected, given that many social marketers see their basic product as information, or they see social marketing as working primarily through channels of communication with information as its primary resource (Young 1989). However, in commercial marketing, the use of mass media is only one component of the total marketing process. A product also must be designed to meet the buyer's 'needs'; it must be packaged and priced appropriately; it must be easily accessible; it should be 'trial-able' (if a large commitment is required); intermediaries such as wholesalers and retailers must be established; and, where relevant, sales staff must be informed and trained. Only after all these factors are in place are the mass media used to make potential buyers:

- aware of the product,
- aware of the product's benefits,
- aware of where it can be purchased, and
- interested (i.e. motivated) to seek further information, or to purchase or trial the product.

In the same way, a campaign that aims to promote health through encouraging individual behaviour change must be based on more than just mass media. Programs and strategies are required at community level (i.e. they must be accessible); the activities promoted must be 'do-able' (i.e. within the target group's capacities) or learn-able (i.e. skills must be defined and training must be available for specific activities); and they must be affordable. Social marketing, by definition, is a far more comprehensive and effective approach than simply using television advertising. It is little wonder therefore that many health promotion campaigns that have relied solely on mass media have failed to have any lasting effect.

Case study 5.1

Social marketing and drink-driving-related crashes

A systematic review of the effectiveness of mass media-supported campaigns for reducing alcohol-impaired driving (AID) and alcohol-related crashes was recently conducted in the USA. In eight studies that met the criteria for inclusion in the review, the median decrease in alcohol-related crashes resulting from the campaigns was 13 per cent. Economic analyses of campaign effects indicated that the benefits to society were greater than the costs. The mass media-supported campaigns reviewed were generally carefully planned and well executed, attained adequate audience exposure, and were implemented in conjunction with other ongoing prevention activities, such as high-visibility enforcement. Hence there is strong evidence that, under these conditions, social marketing campaigns are effective in reducing AID and alcohol-related crashes.

Elder et al. 2004

Principles and practices of social marketing

A number of aspects of marketing have been discussed in the context of social marketing (Donovan & Henley 2003; Donovan & Owen 1994). Those most relevant for health promotion are the following: the marketing concept; the concept of exchange; customer value; market segmentation; competition and the principle of differential advantage; the use of market research; and the integration of the planning process. These concepts are discussed below.

1. The marketing concept: a consumer orientation

A customer focus is the essence of a marketing approach. Marketers seek profits or increased levels of participation in an activity or service through the identification of customer needs, the development of products and services to meet these needs, and the pricing, packaging, promotion and distribution of these products in accordance with consumer habits, aspirations and expectations.

A basic distinction between social and commercial marketing is that social marketing usually is not based on needs experienced by consumers but on needs identified by health experts. However, a marketing approach emphasises that the development, delivery and promotion of the health message and products or services must be carried out in accordance with consumers' needs. For example, messages about immunisation must be in a language consumers understand, the promised benefits must be relevant, and the messages must be placed in media that consumers attend to.

2. The concept of exchange

The concept of exchange has long been described as the core concept of marketing: marketing is the exchange that takes place between consuming groups and supplying groups.

The essential factor that differentiates exchanges from other forms of need satisfaction is that each party to the exchange both gains and receives value. At the same time, each party perceives the offerings to involve costs. Hence it is the ratio of the perceived benefits to the costs that determines choice between alternatives (Kotler & Andreasen 1987). Kotler (1988) lists the following as necessary conditions for the potential for exchange:

1. There are at least two parties.
2. Each party offers something that might be of value to the other party.
3. Each party is capable of communication and delivery.
4. Each party is free to accept or reject the offer.
5. Each party believes it is appropriate or desirable to deal with the other party.

The lessons for social marketers are that we must offer something perceived to be of value to our target audiences and recognise that consumers must outlay resources, such as time, money, physical comfort, lifestyle changes or psychological effort, in exchange for the promised benefits. It also means that we must offer something of value to intermediaries, such as GPs, pharmacists and others whom we wish to involve in interventions.

3. Customer value: the concept of the marketing mix

There are two basic concepts with respect to customer value. First, customers do not just buy products or services, they buy benefits, or bundles of benefits.

Case study 5.2

Target marketing for health checks

As part of a project to encourage men to visit their doctor for a check-up, the Cancer Council of Western Australia ad below was placed in the sporting news section of the daily newspaper, occupied half a page and had a 'male interest' headline to attract attention. The advertisement included a self-assessment questionnaire to attract readers to the content of the ad and, it was hoped, to trigger some action if the score indicated that action was required. This approach was based on research which suggested that men like to have health feedback in the nature of a score. A telephone number was included to provide further information to those who called.

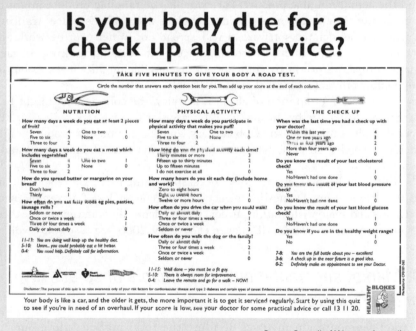

Cancer Council of Western Australia

Charles Revson of Revlon said, 'In the factory we make cosmetics; in the store we sell hope.' Others have made the point that although someone might buy a quarter-inch drill (the product), what they want (the benefit) is a quarter-inch hole (Kotler 1988).

Second, the 'four Ps' of the marketing mix all contribute to customer value. The four Ps are: product (brand name and reputation; packaging and so on), price (monetary cost; credit terms and so on), promotion (advertising;

sales promotion; publicity and public relations; personal selling), and place or distribution (i.e. physical distribution, number and type of outlets; opening hours; atmosphere in outlets; availability of public transport; availability and ease of parking). The marketing manager's task is to blend these four elements so as to provide maximal value to particular market segments. For example time and effort costs are reduced by making the product easily obtainable (e.g. wide distribution; vending machines in appropriate locations); trial-able before commitment (e.g. sample packs; in office/in-home demonstrations; 'seven days free trial'); easy to pay for (e.g. credit card acceptance; lay-by; hire purchase); and easy to use (e.g. user friendly packaging; instructions on use; free training courses).

A concept that ties these two aspects (customer benefits and the four Ps) together is Kotler's (1988) concept of the core product, the augmented product and the actual tangible product. For example the tangible product might be a computer. The augmented product involves after-sales service, training, warranties, associated software, a widespread consumer user network and so on. The core product is better management decision making. In fact, many companies primarily compete not on tangible product features but on augmented product features (Levitt 1969).

In the health promotion of physical activity, the core product might be a longer, healthier life by means of cardiovascular disease risk reduction, the actual product might be an aerobics class, and the augmented product might include a crèche, off-peak discount rates, clean hygienic change rooms and a complimentary towel.

A fifth P—People—applies to services, something particularly appropriate in health promotion. Domestic violence helpline counsellors, for example, need extensive and appropriate training to deal with violent callers and encourage them to join perpetrator programs (Donovan et al. 1999, 2000; see case study 5.3).

4. Market segmentation: the principle of selectivity and concentration

Market segmentation involves dividing the total market into groups of individuals that are more like each other than like individuals in other groups. The fundamental issue is to identify groups that will respond to different products or marketing strategies and, for commercial organisations, to select and concentrate on those segments in which the organisation can be most competitive.

The segmentation process has three phases:

1. dividing the total market into segments and developing profiles of these segments
2. evaluating each segment and selecting one or more segments as target markets

Case study 5.3

The Freedom From Fear campaign marketing mix

The Western Australian Freedom From Fear campaign encourages violent and potentially violent men to call a Men's Domestic Violence Helpline where counsellors attempt to persuade the callers to enrol in counselling programs. The primary medium for reaching violent and potentially violent men is television advertising (especially in sporting programs), supported by radio advertising and posters. Extensive formative research was undertaken to ensure acceptance of the advertisement messages by the target group without negatively affecting victims, children and relevant stakeholders.

The helpline is staffed by counsellors (people specifically trained to deal with violent men), who are able to assess callers and conduct lengthy telephone counselling (i.e. product) with members of the target audience. Anonymity is assured, and there is no pressure on men. The primary aim of the helpline counsellors is to refer as many as callers possible into no-fee (i.e. price) government-funded counselling programs provided primarily by private sector organisations in twelve locations throughout the state (i.e. place). This pricing strategy is necessary to ensure that victims of low-income perpetrators would not be disadvantaged by their partner's limited income. Programs were time scheduled (i.e. place) to allow employed men access to programs in non-working hours (i.e. consumer orientation).

The core product—that is, the end benefit being offered to violent men in relationships in exchange for their acceptance of counselling—is the opportunity to keep their relationship (or family) intact by ending the violence towards their partner (and its effect on children). Other products included self-help booklets providing tips on how to control violence and how to contact service providers. These are also provided on audio-cassettes for men with poor reading skills (i.e. consumer orientation).

Donovan & Henley 2004

3. developing a detailed marketing mix (i.e. the 4Ps) for each of the selected segments.

The concept of market segmentation is fundamental to developing communication campaigns and is dealt with in detail below.

Segmentation for health promotion

One of the basic distinctions between health promotion campaigns and commercial marketing campaigns is that health promotion campaigns are usually based not on needs experienced by consumers but on needs identified by health experts or government health authorities (Sirgy et al. 1985). This often leads to a lack of segmentation of an audience and hence a scattergun approach to delivering a message. A focus on consumer or client needs naturally calls for a segmentation of the prospective audience since it is obvious that vastly different subgroups exist in a population, that the differences occur in a variety of dimensions (or bases), and that different strategies and approaches are necessary to reach and communicate effectively with these different subgroups.

Case study 5.4

Targeting by risk factor status

Skin cancer

Have you been checked?

The .... LIONS CLUB has organised a FREE skin cancer screening. Specialists from the LIONS CANCER INSTITUTE will be available to examine people who feel they are at risk of having skin cancer.

If you are 16 years of age or older and have one or more of the following:

- a family member who has had a malignant melanoma
- five or more moles (not freckles) on your arms
- previously had moles or skin cancer removed
- a mole or freckle that is changing size or colour
- fair skin that burns rather than tans
- had blistering sunburn as a child
- any inflamed skin sores that do not heal

then please phone .... to make an appointment.

Venue: ....
Date: ....

If you are concerned but cannot attend the screening on that date, please express your interest with the LIONS CANCER INSTITUTE and see your family doctor.

For health promotion campaigns, target groups often are described in terms of risk factors (e.g. smokers, the obese, the inactive, heavy drinkers, diabetics and so on) or demographic groupings that epidemiologically appear to be at higher risk (e.g. blue-collar groups, sedentary occupations, Aborigines, street kids and so on). Regardless of the base(s) chosen for the initial segmentation (e.g. age and sex), the segments are also usually described or profiled on as many other variables as possible, so as to better understand the chosen segment(s). However, we consider that two fundamental segmentation approaches are useful in social marketing health campaigns: stage segmentation, and attitude and/or behaviour segmentation. These are useful segmentations because the campaign strategies follow directly from the underlying segmentation model.

A stage approach to segmentation: the Prochaska model

A segmentation model directly applicable for much health promotion derives from James Prochaska's clinical work with cigarette and drug addiction (Prochaska & DiClemente 1984, 1986). This model now forms the basis of some social marketing frameworks (Andreasen 1995).

Prochaska divides the total target segment (e.g. smokers) into subsegments depending on their stage in progression towards adoption of a desired type of behaviour (i.e. quitting smoking).

Prochaska and DiClemente's (1984) stages are:

1. *precontemplation*—where the individual is not even considering modifying their unhealthy behaviour
2. *contemplation*—where the individual is considering changing unhealthy behaviour, but not in the immediate future
3. *preparation*—where the individual plans to try to change their unhealthy behaviour in the immediate future (i.e. in the next two weeks or appropriate time frame)
4. *action*—the immediate (six-month) period following trial and adoption of the recommended behaviour and cessation of the unhealthy behaviour
5. *maintenance*—the period following the action stage until the unhealthy behaviour is fully extinguished
6. *termination*—when the problem behaviour is completely eliminated; that is, zero temptation across all problem situations.

Donovan and Owen (1994) claim that mass media health promotion campaigns are most influential in the precontemplation and contemplation stages (by raising the salience and personal relevance of the issue), of moderate influence in the preparation stage (by reinforcing perceptions of self-efficacy and maintaining salience of the perceived benefits of adopting the recommended behaviour), and of least influence in the action and maintenance stages, where beliefs and attitudes are well established and where socioenvironmental influences on the achieved behaviour are greatest.

A number of studies have shown that different message and intervention strategies are more or less appropriate for people in the different stages (Prochaska et al. 1994). For example Donovan, Leivers and Hannaby (1997) showed that precontemplating smokers reacted differently to a set of anti-smoking advertisements relative to contemplating smokers.

Attitude–behaviour segmentation: the Sheth–Frazier model

Sheth and Frazier (1982) developed a model of strategy mix choice for behaviour change. They suggest that there are four major processes of planned social change, each one most appropriate for each of four combinations of attitude–behaviour consistency or discrepancy (see table 5.1).

Table 5.1: A typology of strategy mix for planned social change (Sheth & Frazier 1982)

| | ATTITUDE | |
	Positive	Negative
Perform	Cell 1 Reinforcement process	Cell 2 Rationalisation process Attitude change
DESIRED BEHAVIOUR		
Don't perform	Cell 3 Inducement process Behaviour change	Cell 4 Confrontation process

Survey data provides the proportion of the population of interest in each of these cells, with the cell designation indicating the appropriate strategy for each cell. That is, when attitudes and behaviour are consistent and in the desired direction with respect to the relevant behaviour (cell 1), a reinforcement process is called for to sustain the desired behaviour. This can be done by (a) reinforcing the attitude, (b) reinforcing the behaviour, or both. For example people who are both predisposed towards exercise and carry out regular exercise can be encouraged to continue to do so by reminding them of the benefits of exercise or by making it easier to carry out.

If attitudes are positive but the behaviour is not being performed (cell 3), an inducement process aimed at minimising or removing organisational, socioeconomic, time and place constraints (such as improving availability of exercise facilities) should be used.

Where the behaviour is being performed but the attitude is negative (cell 2), rationalisation is most appropriate (e.g. relating exercise to good health). Where attitudes are negative and the behaviour is not being performed (cell 4), confrontation might be the answer (e.g. a face-to-face warning by a GP to an individual of the health risks of not taking any exercise).

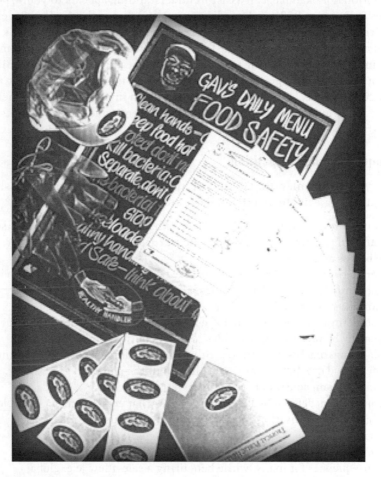

Materials promoting good hygiene for food handlers in North Queensland as part of Queensland's Health Foodsafe Campaign

5. Competition and the principle of differential advantage

In marketing, competition and differential advantage refer to an analysis of the marketer's resources versus those of the competition, with the aim of determining where the company enjoys a differential advantage over the opposition. In a wider sense it relates to monitoring and understanding competitive activity, sometimes to emulate or follow such activity, in other cases to pre-empt or counter competitors' activities.

In health promotion, it is necessary to identify, understand and develop counter-strategies for the competition. A study of alcohol advertising and promotion, for example, can assist in understanding appeals to young people (Jones & Donovan 2001) and for identifying breaches of the Alcohol Beverages Advertising Code (Jones & Donovan 2002). Similarly, advocacy groups need to monitor such industries as the tobacco and food industries and attempt to pre-empt industry marketing tactics that have a negative influence on children and other vulnerable groups. For example many non-nutritious snack foods offer convenience, low price, good taste and a fun image. To compete, healthy snack foods must satisfy these same needs, or introduce 'new' benefits that are attractive to people.

Categorising the competition

Donovan and Henley (2003) propose the following categories to assist in designing strategies to monitor and counter the competition:

- competitors clearly defined by the fact that any use of their products is harmful (e.g. tobacco use; some illicit drugs; leaded petrol; some forms of asbestos and so on)
- competitors defined by the fact that excess use or abuse of their products is harmful (e.g. some illicit drugs; alcohol; guns; motor vehicles; gambling and so on)
- competitors defined by beliefs and values that inhibit the uptake of healthy behaviour (e.g. attitudes to birth control inhibiting family planning; machismo attitudes inhibiting condom use and facilitating the spread of AIDS), or affect the health of the planet in general (e.g. materialism; consumption as lifestyle)
- competitors defined by beliefs and values that create conflict in society (e.g. racist organisations; fundamentalist religious organisations; terrorist groups)
- competitors defined by beliefs and values that have negative consequences for many, while benefiting a select few (e.g. global corporations; privatisation of government services; armaments suppliers; media organisations).

6. The use of market research

Given all of the above, it should be apparent that effective marketing is a research-based process. Research in social marketing is concerned both with epidemiological data and with assessment of such factors as: what health 'products' (e.g. exercise, dietary fat reduction, smoking cessation and so on) does the community perceive as priorities for action; what tangible products can be developed to facilitate the adoption of health-promoting behaviour or to reduce risk (e.g. no tar cigarettes, low-fat foods, quit smoking kits, exercise videos and so on); what programs or services can be offered (e.g. weight control, aerobics classes, educational videos on the benefits of exercise; training videos on how to institute worksite programs); how the message strategy should be developed; what social and structural facilitators and inhibitors need to be taken into account; who are the relevant influencers and intermediaries; which media (television, radio, press) and which media vehicles (specific programs), if any, can be used to reach the target audience(s) cost-effectively; and what activities are being undertaken by 'anti-health' marketers.

7. An integrated planning process

The marketing process is an integrated process such that elements of the marketing mix, the organisation's resources, the use of market research, and the selection and concentration on specific market segments are all combined to maximise the value of the organisation's offerings to the consumer, and hence profit to the company. For health organisations, this might translate to intended changes in knowledge, attitude or behaviour.

This integration strongly implies the need for a systematic strategic planning process: the setting of clearly defined overall goals; the setting of measurable objectives to meet the overall goals; the delineation of strategies and tactics to achieve these objectives; and management and feedback systems to ensure that the plan is implemented as desired, to avert or deal with problems as they arise.

Differences between commercial and social marketing: can we sell health like we sell soap?

Although the principles and practices of marketing are clearly applicable to the promotion of healthy lifestyles, it is a mistake to assume that social marketing is similar to commercial marketing in all respects. Even within marketing, different approaches are more or less appropriate for different products. In short, although some of the principles of marketing are applicable, selling health or any other socially desirable product cannot be fully equated with selling soap.

Bloom and Novelli (1981) and Rothschild (1979) list a number of important differences between the marketing of commercial products and social marketing. The major differences are:

1. Commercial products tend to offer instant gratification whereas the benefits of healthy behaviour are often delayed.
2. Social marketing attempts to replace undesirable behaviour with behaviour that is often more costly in time or effort and, at least in the short term, less pleasurable or in fact unpleasant.

3. Commercial marketing mostly aims at groups already positive towards the product and its benefits, whereas social marketing often is directed towards hard-to-reach, at-risk groups who are often most antagonistic to change.
4. Health risk behaviour is often extremely complex, both at a personal and at a social level, and far more so than the behaviour involved in purchasing most commercial products.
5. Intermediaries in commercial marketing are far fewer in type and generally far easier to deal with (although perhaps more costly) than in social marketing.
6. Defining and communicating the product is far more difficult in social marketing, especially where different experts might have different views on the subject.
7. The exchange process is far easier to define in commercial marketing than in social marketing.
8. Much targeted health-related behaviour is inconsistent with social pressures.
9. Ethical questions and issues of equity are far more complex and important (e.g. victim blaming) in social marketing.
10. Social marketing should also be directed towards not just changes in individual behaviour but also changes in systems and social structures that operate to the detriment of the health of populations.

The techniques and principles of marketing are applicable to any consumer decision, yet their effective application to health promotion requires an understanding of both areas. In practical terms this requires close cooperation between marketing experts, public health professionals and, for mass media campaign components, behavioural scientists with expertise in communication theory and attitude and behaviour change.

Using the media

Some community focus strategies are generated from within the community (i.e. community development). Community organisation (as distinct from community development) involves mobilisation of the community in line with the needs deemed appropriate by health authorities. Mass media strategies are also more intrusive, with programs being imposed on the community as a whole, rather than being generated by individual demand within a community. Still, the requirements of a successful media message are the same: it must have individual appeal that encourages the individual to act. According to one media expert:

Message begins with 'me'. Me singular. Indeed there is no such thing, really, as mass communication. It's a contradiction in terms. Communication is an intensely personal one-to-one process, whether you are doing it over the telephone or over the television network. Uni—uno, one—is the very heart of comm-uni-cation. (Bevins 1988)

The influence of the media in health promotion has been hotly debated in the past. Although they have been used for some time in a range of health and public service programs, the media have been looked at seriously only since the early 1970s. Since then it has become accepted that well-designed and implemented mass media campaigns based on sound communication principles and developed with close cooperation between health and media professionals can have substantial impact, both in the health area and in other social areas (e.g. see Egger et al. 1993; Donovan & Leivers 1993; Reid 1996; Elder et al. 1996; Pierce et al. 1990).

The components of the media can be classified in a number of different ways: broadcast versus print, visual versus auditory and so on. For the current analysis, 'media' will be defined as mass reach, meaning those with a more impersonal general distribution (e.g. TV, radio, press, magazines), and limited reach, meaning those with a more personal distribution and limited communications intent (e.g. posters, pamphlets, T shirts, bumper stickers and so on).

Media might or might not be used as part of other community focus strategies such as social marketing, community organisation and community development.

A summary of media approaches covered in this section is shown in table 5.2 on page 114. Community organisation and community development approaches will be covered in chapter 6.

Mass media methods

The three major methods of using the media in the previous edition of this book were advertising, publicity and 'edutainment'. Following Donovan and Henley (2003), we add web sites and civic journalism as two methods worthy of increasing attention in health promotion.

Advertising

'Advertising' refers to the paid placement of messages in various media vehicles by an identified source. We include here the voluntary placement by the media of social change messages that are clearly in the form of paid advertisements (called community or public service announcements: CSAs or PSAs).

Publicity

'Publicity' refers to the unpaid placement of messages in the media, usually in news or current affairs programs, but also in feature articles or documentaries. Publicity involves persuading the media to run a particular story or cover a particular event in a way that creates, maintains or increases the target audience's awareness of or favourable attitudes towards the organisation's

Table 5.2: A summary of media methods

Type	Characteristics
Limited reach media	
Pamphlets	Information transmission. Best where cognition rather than emotion is desired outcome.
Information sheets	Quick convenient information. Use as series with storage folder. Not for complex behaviour change.
Newsletters	Continuity. Personalised. Labour-intensive, and requires detailed commitment and needs assessment before commencing.
Posters	Agenda-setting function. Visual message. Creative input required. Possibility of graffiti might be considered.
T-shirts	Emotive. Personal. Useful for cementing attitudes and commitment to program/idea.
Stickers	Short messages to identify/motivate the user and cement commitment. Cheap, persuasive.
Videos	Instructional. Motivational. Useful for personal viewing with adults as back-up to other programs.
DVDs and CDs	Provides the opportunity for portable, attractive, easy to use, multimedia transmitted information
Mass reach media	
Television	Awareness, arousal, modelling and image creation role. May be increasingly useful in information and skills training as awareness and interest in health increases.
Radio	Informative, interactive (talkback). Cost-effective and useful in creating awareness, providing information.
Newspapers	Long and short copy information. Material dependent on type of paper and day of week.
Magazines	Wide readership and influence. Useful as supportive role and to inform and provide social proof.
Internet	Can serve a wide role from personal information transmission to group sessions to 'blogging'.

products or message, or towards the organisation itself. Many campaigns now involve press conferences with celebrities and staged events, supported by such activities as providing the media with press releases, videotapes, feature articles and photographs, and by making experts available for interview on radio and television.

Edutainment

A third and increasing use of the media for health promotion is the deliberate inclusion of socially desirable messages in entertainment vehicles, such as television soap operas, to achieve social change objectives. For example the Harvard alcohol project in the USA asked television writers to introduce into top-rated TV programs actions and themes that would reinforce and encourage a social norm that drivers don't drink (DeJong & Winsten 1990).

Civic journalism

Rosen (1994) describes civic (or public) journalism as

> an unfolding philosophy about the place of the journalist in public life [that] has emerged most clearly in recent initiatives in the newspaper world that show journalists trying to connect with their communities ... by encouraging civic participation or regrounding the coverage of politics in the imperatives of public discussion and debate.

Whereas standard journalism thrives on conflict and disagreement, civic journalism attempts to build community consensus and cooperation; whereas standard journalism seeks to emphasise differences and seek interviews with those known to have extremely opposing views on a topic, civic journalism emphasises similarities and seeks to emphasise more moderate views.

Case study 5.5

Civic journalism: the *Akron Beacon Journal*'s race relations project

Following race riots in Los Angeles, the *Akron Beacon Journal* instituted a year-long series of articles, entitled 'A question of colour', dealing with five issues: racial attitudes, housing, education, economic status and crime. Each topic was presented over three or four consecutive days, covering several pages each day, and including a number of graphics and people photos. The amount of space devoted to the series was a clear indicator to the reader of the importance placed on the issue by the newspaper.

The articles contained a mix of statistical information (e.g. percentage of home ownership by colour, percentage occupational status by colour and so on); traditional journalism reporting and interpretation of past and current events; the identification of major changes and non-changes over the decades; reports on the results of focus groups among both blacks and whites that probed beliefs and attitudes held by the two groups towards each other (and post-group interviews with participants); and reports on survey research of the extent to which people in the community held various beliefs and attitudes. Right from the start, the *Journal*'s readers were invited to 'Tell us what you think' about race relations and 'how blacks and whites can better understand each other', by faxing, phoning or writing to the newspaper. The newspaper periodically printed readers' contributions. This involvement of the community evolved into the 'Coming Together' community project, which continued after the Question of Colour series finished in December 1993.

Donovan & Henley 2003

Web sites and interactive information technology

The arrival of the Internet has increased the average individual's access to information and, for certain marketers, has provided a sales channel without which they could not have reached markets other than their small geographical catchment areas. However, it has not increased the public's ability to interpret information, or to judge the reliability and validity of the information provided. This unfettered access to the web increases the need for credible pro-social organisations not only to have a strong presence on the web but also to continue to position themselves in the public eye as the credible, authoritative sources for information in their areas.

For health promoters, the web provides a relatively efficient and inexpensive forum for the dissemination of information and materials (e.g. see www. comminit.com and www.toolsofchange.com).

Donovan and Henley list the following 'new media' developments with implications for social marketers and health promoters:

- *Electronic communities*: where all households, retailers, businesses, schools, health and welfare organisations in a particular geographic (usually local government) area are given access to each other (and each other's products and services) via an intranet. The opportunities for 'direct emailing', marketing promotions and information dissemination are clearly enormous, although the potential for information overload is also high.
- *Multimedia and interactive technology*: multimedia PCs are those with digital audio and a CD-ROM player and hence can show pictures, sound, text and graphics. Newer versions of the CD, such as the DVD (digital versatile disc, or digital video disc), will not only store far more but also have far greater capabilities. Multimedia PC developments provide opportunities for elaborate message execution (e.g. combining messages from celebrities, film clips, computer-generated animations, demonstrations and so on).

Interactivity is concerned with mutual responsiveness (Postma 1999). At this stage, most opportunities for interactivity are via web sites and CD-ROMs, although comprehensive interactive TV will add a new (visual) dimension to that currently offered by computers.

Many health organisations have developed interactive web sites where visitors can, for example, answer a questionnaire about their dietary habits and receive an immediate diagnosis and prognosis about dietary changes. Anti-tobacco campaigners are developing similar methods that classify smokers according to their stage of change, and then present messages tailored to the smoker's stage of change and other characteristics.

Case study 5.6

Interactive web sites: the USA's National Youth Anti-Drug Media Campaign

This campaign brings together a number of interactive web sites aimed at youth, parents, teachers, media personnel and other stakeholders, placing messages on a variety of partners' web sites, placing advertising on consumer web sites and with a major Internet service provider (AOL, America On Line), and developing messages and programs for leading child and parent news content sites. One partnership includes a deal with Marvel Comic Books that produces a special Spider-Man comic book series (downloadable from the web) teaching kids anti-drug messages and media literacy skills for deconstructing what they see and hear in movies, television and popular songs.

Schwartz 2000; from Donovan & Henley 2003

Choosing media methods

The decision about whether to use advertising, publicity, edutainment, web sites or interactive media, or civic journalism, or some combination of these in any health promotion campaign is determined by a number of factors, including the objectives of the campaign, the budget, the relative effectiveness of the different modes in reaching and influencing the target audiences, the complexity of the message, time constraints, relations with the media, and the nature and types of media and media vehicles available.

From the campaign manager's perspective, the primary advantages of paid advertising relate to control factors; that is, control over message content, message exposure—timing and location, and hence target audience, and frequency of exposure. Control over message content not only allows precise specification of the informational content of the message but also allows the creation of imagery and the use of various message executional techniques and appeals that enhance the persuasive power of the message.

Advertising's major disadvantage is cost. However, because the number of people exposed to advertising is usually quite large, the cost per individual contact and impact is often low, especially relative to face-to-face methods.

Publicity shares the ability of advertising to reach large numbers of people in a relatively short period of time, but has the disadvantage of less control over message content, message exposure and frequency (unless the issue is sufficiently newsworthy to attract continuing coverage for several days). A press release, for example, might be rewritten in a way that omits or distorts crucial information, be relegated to the later pages of a newspaper, appear only in a very late TV or radio news spot, or even be totally ignored. On the other hand, publicity is generally perceived as more credible than paid advertising (because the source is presumably unbiased, or less biased), and is less costly. However, costs are incurred in developing materials, staging events and so on, and often there are fees for engaging professional public relations agencies.

Edutainment also has the ability to reach large numbers of people in a relatively short period of time, but has the disadvantages of reduced control over message content. The primary advantage of edutainment is the ability to attract the attention of people who might otherwise deliberately avoid messages that appear in an obvious educational form. Where a health authority or sponsoring body is not directly involved in producing the show, edutainment can be done economically. If a show is a commercial success, the health organisation could even earn a profit (Coleman & Meyer 1990).

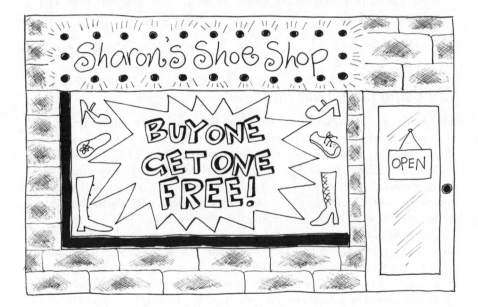

Web sites are now almost an expected part of any health promotion initiative. Useful web sites allow the audience access to information about an issue and stakeholders access to program information. Interactive elements can be built into the site, as well as links established to other sites. Web site design becomes expensive when interactive elements are included, but the major issues are maintaining and updating the site. Sites are often established in a burst of enthusiasm but become quickly neglected and dated.

Civic journalism is useful for complex issues that require extensive information to be absorbed in a non-emotive atmosphere. As Donovan and Henley (2003) point out, the major difficulty in Australia is that there is no established tradition of civic journalism; newspapers appear to be focused on advertising revenue rather than on quality journalism, and hence individual journalists have little support from their editors and publishers.

Roles of the media in health promotion campaigns

There appear to be three major roles, two of which primarily apply to the targeting of individual behaviour change and one to the achievement of sociopolitical objectives.

Targeting individual behaviour change

According to Donovan (1991), the two primary communication objectives for most campaigns are to inform (or educate) and to persuade (or motivate).

The distinction between these two roles is blurred in that the provision of information is generally not intended for its own sake, but is usually meant to lead to desired behaviour changes. However, although information alone can arouse emotions and motivate some people to cease an unhealthy practice, it is clear from the public health literature that information in itself is insufficient to bring about desired behaviour changes in most individuals.

Targeting sociopolitical change: media advocacy

Most uses of the mass media in health promotion have been directed towards change of risk behaviour at the individual level. However, the mass media also have been used to advocate, in order to achieve sociopolitical environmental changes that affect health (Chapman & Lupton 1994). Advocacy for health promotion is a relatively ill-defined process with broad general characteristics, summed up by Chapman (2004) as being:

1. a focus on 'upstream' goals
2. goals that are invariably contested, and
3. methods that are opportunistic and responsive.

The quit smoking lobby is to date the most professional health advocacy group successfully using media advocacy. It has used the media to redefine smoking as a public health issue of concern to all, and to attack the morals and motives of tobacco companies' marketing techniques. The subsequent arousal of public opinion has been used to support direct lobbying of legislative changes, such as restricting the advertising of cigarettes and the sponsorship of sporting and arts events by tobacco companies. Advocacy often has as its primary outcome a change in the physical environment (e.g. protests for better roads). However, in achieving such an outcome, it generally aims initially at changing the sociocultural environment. Other areas in which advocacy has worked effectively are drink-driving, sports injury prevention, AIDS/HIV control and nutrition advertising, giving rise to several publications that outline processes and practices of advocacy (Wallack et al. 1993; Chapman & Lupton 1994; Siegal & Doner 1998).

Table 5.3 shows that each of these methods—advertising, publicity and edutainment—can be utilised in conjunction with any of these overall objectives: educate, motivate and advocate.

Table 5.3: A framework for using media in social marketing

Ways of using the media

	Advertising	Publicity	Edutainment	Web sites	Civic journalism
Objectives					
Educate	**	**	****	*****	****
Motivate	****	**	****	**	***
Advocate	***	***	**	**	****

Both individual and sociopolitical change objectives should be combined for any comprehensive health campaign. However, in some cases it is likely that campaigns targeted at individuals must first have some influence on beliefs and attitudes towards the recommended behaviour before sociopolitical advocacy objectives can be achieved. For example it is unlikely that efforts to frame smoking as a public health issue would have been as successful without prior QUIT campaigns that emphasised the ill-health effects of smoking. Similarly, efforts to control smoking indoors undoubtedly were facilitated by increasing awareness of the health effects of passive smoking.

There are a number of objectives that can be classified under the three overall roles of information, motivation or persuasion, and advocacy, which are discussed below. However, it should be noted that the classification is not mutually exclusive.

Informational objectives

- Informing (or educating) people about the negative health effects of smoking and passive smoking, and the positive health effects of cessation and smoke-free areas.
- Clarifying misperceptions and/or confusion that people might have about various health effects of smoking.
- Reminding people of the positive and negative health effects of which they are already aware and maintaining the salience of this knowledge.
- Directing people to information on where and how to get help, or how to help themselves.
- Informing the target audience of specific events ('15 June is Quit Day'), or programs and services ('Quit classes, 3pm daily, St Bernard's Hall').

Motivational or persuasion objectives

- Reinforcing non-smokers or ex-smokers, especially recent quitters.
- Generating emotional arousal to increase people's motivations to quit smoking.
- Sensitising or predisposing individuals to other contributory influences (arguably the major role as a facilitator of behaviour change), such as family pressures to quit or availability of assistance to quit.
- Increasing awareness of both prescriptive and, where appropriate, popular norms (Cialdini 1984), and hence providing social support for those who wish to quit.
- Stimulating word-of-mouth communications about the health issues in question and hence encouraging peer (and other) group discussion and decision making—a very important role for the diffusion of social issues.

Advocacy-related objectives

- Increasing community awareness of smoking as a public health issue; that is, placing the issue on the community's agenda, or 'agenda setting'.
- Creating or increasing community awareness of a particular point of view with respect to passive smoking; that is, framing the community agenda.

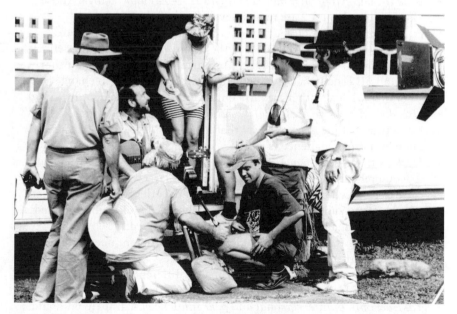

Singer John Williamson shown in production of a TV advertisement to prevent dengue fever in North Queensland

Queensland Health

- Creating or maintaining a favourable attitude towards such issues as restrictions on tobacco promotion, smoke free entertainment venues and so on.
- Creating a view that the issue is a sufficiently serious one for community concern; that is, legitimising the issue.
- Generating a positive community mood within which health authority policies, including research and regulatory measures, such as banning of sponsorship by tobacco companies, can be introduced with minimal opposition and/or maximal support.

Components of successful media campaigns

A number of researchers, both in health promotion and in communications, have attempted to identify the conditions in which the media is most effective in promoting health. Distilling a number of reviews and other research leads to the following practical recommendations for designing a successful campaign:

- *Carry out formative research.* Intuition is not a sufficient basis on which to devise a campaign. Materials should be developed from skilled formative research (i.e. focus groups, surveys), pre-tested and evaluated during exposure.
- *Base the campaign on a model of attitude–behaviour change.* Those discussed in chapter 2 are most relevant for health promotion.
- *Fully understand the topic being communicated.* Some topics are difficult and complex to teach (e.g. the nature of drugs and their effects), whereas others might be easily communicated (e.g. hygiene). Similarly, certain well-established types of behaviour are difficult to change (e.g. smoking), whereas others require only a minor effort (e.g. not littering).
- *Use skilled creative personnel.* Determining a message is simple. Executing that message in a way that is optimally received and acted upon by a target audience is a highly skilled process.
- *Understand the audience.* The extent to which a message is attended to, comprehended and used by an audience is largely determined by the extent to which the messenger understands the audience. Detailed profiles of an audience need to be established as a preliminary to media development if a message is to be optimally received.
- *Target the message.* Different subgroups have different needs, interests, beliefs and attitudes. Hence, different messages—or at least different message executions—should be tailored to different groups. Different groups could be reached through different channels.
- *Take account of interpersonal and peer influences.* Campaigns should attempt to stimulate interpersonal contact, such as the promotion of group and community activities and the activation of interpersonal communication networks.

- *Optimise contact with the message.* This doesn't mean total bombardment. Research indicates that concentrated bursts of spot messages often work better than the same quantity of messages strung out over a long period.
- *Use multiple channels.* Multiple communication channels (i.e. different media and media vehicles plus various non-media channels) tend to have a synergistic effect, are mutually reinforcing and can carry different types of information.
- *Use a credible source or spokesperson.* Source credibility is a major factor affecting message acceptance. Spokespersons are often assumed to be credible to the target audience; for example the use of celebrities and sport stars in anti-drug promotions to youth is common practice, yet research suggests that youth identify only with certain aspects of an idealised role model, such as their ability to play music, sport and so on. If other aspects (e.g. their attitude to drugs) conflict with overwhelming peer pressure, the model will be discarded rather than the anti-social habit. Testing source credibility is essential in pre-testing the message.
- *Set realistic goals and a realistic duration for the study.* Major shifts in behaviour are not common in large populations over short periods. Hence it is important that intermediate goals, such as knowledge and attitudinal changes, are set rather than behavioural goals. Also, ongoing campaigns are necessary to maintain awareness and to reinforce attitude and behaviour change. Furthermore, many campaigns set large, unrealistic changes as their criteria for success (e.g. reducing alcoholism) rather than more realistic immediate changes (e.g. reducing drink-driving).
- *Provide environmental supports for change.* Research has shown consistently that most media campaigns require 'on-the-ground' back-up support for optimum effect. To accomplish this, media should be accompanied by strategies of community organisation.
- *Ensure that input from a behavioural scientist guides the communications agency.* Commercial agencies need to be guided by behavioural science principles. The danger otherwise is that creative ideas will drive the strategy rather than the strategy driving the creative ideas.

Appropriate situations for media use

Some of the situations in which mass media have been found to be most appropriate are:

- *When wide exposure is desired.* Mass media offer the widest possible exposure, although this might be at some cost. Cost-benefit considerations therefore are at the core of media selection.

- *When the time frame is urgent.* Mass media offer the best opportunity for reaching either large numbers of people or specific target groups within a short time frame.
- *When public discussion is likely to facilitate the educational process.* Media messages can be emotional and thought provoking. Because of the possible breadth of coverage, intrusion can occur at many different levels, stimulating discussion and thereby expanding the influence of a message.
- *When awareness is a main goal.* By their very nature the media are tools for awareness creating. Where awareness of a health issue is important to the resolution of that issue, the mass media can increase awareness quickly and effectively.
- *When media authorities are 'on side'.* Where journalists, editors and programmers are 'on side' with respect to a particular health issue, this often guarantees greater support in terms of space and editorial content.

Hard-to-reach audiences

Some criticism of the use of mass media has centred on the claim that mass media are ineffective in reaching important target groups. In some cases this is a valid criticism in that media campaigns have been directed towards various groups that would have been more effectively targeted via some other method. The question remains whether the media can be used to reach 'hard-to-reach' (HTR) groups and, if so, what roles would they play for these groups?

Hard-to-reach groups are usually defined in terms of their non-responsive-ness to mainstream media campaigns. However, it is important to distinguish between those who are hard to reach because of (1) low access to mainstream media, and those who are hard to reach because of (2) apparent imperviousness to media campaigns. The latter definition is the most used, and accessibility is often included as a correlate of personality and lifestyle factors, such as a distrust of large government organisations, a sense of fatalism and poor cognitive processing skills. We suggest two alternative definitions:

1. hard-to-reach: to refer to those not accessible via media, and
2. hard-to-influence: to refer to those not responsive to messages delivered via the media.

Groups like sex workers, intravenous drug users, street kids and other homeless people, Aboriginal fringe dwellers and non-English-speaking immigrants are generally thought of with respect to accessibility. Yet there is now considerable evidence that such groups are accessible via mainstream media, including ethnic media, although care must be taken in scheduling and vehicle selection.

With respect to both accessibility and responsiveness, the answer lies in carrying out adequate formative research to assess, first, whether a potential target audience is accessible and then, given accessibility, whether it is likely to be responsive to media messages. In some cases, the role of the media might be limited to directing people to other campaign interventions (e.g. telephone information services, interpreter services, needle exchange locations and so on) rather than to belief or attitude change.

Career opportunities in health promotion

Skills in social marketing open up a range of opportunities in the private sector as well as in health promotion and other social services. There are opportunities in marketing, advertising and social research, particularly in qualitative and quantitative processes in market research. Focus group research can be an occupation in itself, with several organisations offering services directly to corporations, media outlets or advertising agencies. Subspecialties in social marketing can include graphic design, health journalism (freelance or employed), merchandising, newsletter production, and web site design and development. The scope is expanding for health promotion personnel to act in a consulting capacity to organisations involved in media and other promotional productions, such as event management.

References

Andreasen, A. R., 1995, *Marketing Social Change: Changing Behaviour to Promote Health, Social Development, and the Environment*, Jossey-Bass, San Francisco.

Bevins, J., 1988, *Third National Drug Educators' Workshop: Workshop Proceedings*, vol. 1, West Australian Department of Health, Perth, WA.

Bloom, P. N., & Novelli, W. D., 1981, 'Problems and challenges of social marketing', *J Market* 45:79–88.

Brownell, K. D., 2004, *Food Fight*, Contemporary Books, NY.

Buchanan, D. R., Reddy, S., & Hossain, Z., 1994, 'Social marketing: a critical appraisal', *Health Prom Int* 9:49–57.

Chapman, S., 2004, 'Public health advocacy', in Moodie, R., & Hulme, A. (eds), *Hands-on Health Promotion*, IP Communications, Melbourne, Vic.

Chapman, S., & Lupton, D., 1994, *The Fight for Public Health: Principles and Practice of Media Advocacy*, BMJ Publishing Group, London.

Cialdini, R. B., 1984, *Influence*, Quill, New York.

Coleman, P. L., & Meyer, R. C. (eds), 1990, *Proceedings from the Enter-Educate Conference: Entertainment for Social Change*, Johns Hopkins University Center for Communication Programs, Baltimore.

DeJong, W., & Winsten, J. A., 1990, 'The use of mass media in substance abuse prevention', *Health Affairs* Summer:30–46.

Donovan, R. J., 1991, 'Public health advertising: execution guidelines for health promotion professionals', *Health Prom J Aust* 1:40–5.

Donovan, R. J., Francas, M., Paterson, D., & Zappelli, R., 2000, 'Formative research for mass media-based campaigns: Western Australia's "Freedom From Fear" campaign targeting male perpetrators of intimate partner violence', *Health Promotion Journal of Australia* 10(2):78–83.

Donovan, R. J., & Henley, N., 2003, *Social Marketing: Principles and Practice*, IP Communications, Melbourne, Vic.

Donovan, R. J., & Leivers, S., 1993, 'Using mass media to change racial stereotype beliefs', *Pub Opin Quart* 57:205–18.

Donovan, R.J., Leivers, S., & Hannaby, L., 1997, *Pre-Contemplators' and Contemplators' Responses to Anti-Smoking Advertising*, Health Promotion Evaluation Unit, University of Western Australia, Perth, WA.

Donovan, R. J., & Owen, N., 1994, 'Social marketing and population interventions', in Dishman, R. K. (ed.), *Advances in Exercise Adherence* (2nd edn), Human Kinetics Publishers, Champaign, Ill.

Donovan, R.J., Paterson, D., & Francas, M., 1999, 'Targeting male perpetrators of intimate partner violence: Western Australia's "Freedom from Fear" campaign', *Social Marketing Quarterly* 5(3):127–43.

Egger, G., Donovan, R. J., & Spark, R., 1993, *Health and the Media: Principles and Practice for Health Promotion*, McGraw-Hill, Sydney.

Elder, J. P., Edwards, C. C., Conway, T. L., Kenney, E., Johnson, C. A., & Bennett, E.D., 1996, 'Independent evaluation of the California Tobacco Education Program', *Public Health Reports* 111:353–8.

Fine, S. H., 1990, *The Marketing of Ideas and Social Issues* (2nd edn), Praeger, New York.

Hastings, G., & Haywood, A., 1994, 'Social marketing: a critical response', *Health Prom Int* 9:59–63.

Hastings, G., McFadyen, L., & Anderson, S., 2000, 'Whose behaviour is it anyway? The broader potential of social marketing', *Social Marketing Quarterly* 6(2):46–58.

Jones, S., & Donovan, R. J., 2001, 'Messages in alcohol advertising targeted to youth', *Australian and New Zealand Journal of Public Health* 25(2):126–31.

—— 2002, 'Self-regulation of alcohol advertising: is it working for Australia?', *J Pub Aff* 2(3):153–65.

Kersh, R., & Morone, J., 2002, 'How the personal becomes political: prohibitions, public health and obesity', *Stud Am Pol Devel* 16:162–75.

Kotler, P., 1988, *Marketing Management: Analysis, Planning, Implementation and Control*, Prentice Hall, Englewood Cliffs, NJ.

Kotler, P., & Andreasen, A. R., 1987, *Strategic Marketing for Nonprofit Organisations*, Prentice Hall, Englewood Cliffs, NJ.

Kotler, P., & Roberto, E. L., 1989, *Social Marketing: Strategies for Changing Public Behaviour*, Free Press, New York.

Kotler, P., & Zaltman, G., 1971, 'Social marketing: an approach to planned social change', *Journal of Marketing* 35:3–12.

Levitt, T., 1969, *The Marketing Mode*, McGraw-Hill, New York.

Lunn, T., 1986, 'Segmenting and constructing markets', in Worcester, R. M., & Downham, J. (eds), *Consumer Market Research Handbook*, North Holland, Amsterdam, pp. 287–424.

Manoff, R. K., 1985, *Social Marketing*, Praeger, New York.

Marketing News, 1985, 'AMA board approves new marketing definition', (1):1.

Nutbeam, D., 1986, 'Health promotion glossary', *Health Promotion* 1(1):113–27.

Pierce, J. P., Macaskill, P., & Hill, D., 1990, 'Long-term effectiveness of mass media-led antismoking campaigns in Australia', *Am J Pub Health* 80(5):565–9.

Postma, P., 1999, *The New Marketing Era*, McGraw-Hill, New York.

Prochaska, J. O., & DiClemente, C. C., 1984, *The Transtheoretical Approach: Crossing the Traditional Boundaries of Therapy*, Dow-Jones/Irwin, Homewood, Ill.

—— 1986, 'Toward a comprehensive model of change', in Miller, W. R., & Heather, N. (eds), *Treating Addictive Behaviours: Processes of Change*, Plenum Press, NY.

Prochaska, J. O., Velicer, W. F., Rossi, J. S., Goldstein, M. G., Marcus, B. H., Rakowski, W., Fiore, C., Harlow, L. L., Redding, C. A., Rosenbloom, D., & Rossi, S. R., 1994, 'Stages of change and decisional balance for 12 problem behaviours', *Health Psych* 13:39–46.

Reid, D., 1996, 'How effective is health education via mass communications?', *Health Ed J* 55:332–44.

Rosen, J., 1994, 'Public journalism: first principles', in Rosen, J., & Merritt Jr, D. (eds), *Public Journalism: Theory and Practice*, Kettering Foundation, Dayton.

Ross, H. S., & Mico, P. R., 1980, *Theory and Practice in Health Education*, Mayfield Publishing Co., Palo Alto, Calif.

Rothschild, M. L., 1979, 'Marketing communications in non-business situations or why it's so hard to sell brotherhood like soap', *J Market* 43:11–20.

Schwartz, B., 1995, *Social Marketing Workshop*, Academy for Educational Development, Washington, DC.

—— 2000, *Fact Sheet: Interactive Program*, Fleishman Hillard, Washington, DC.

Sheth, J. N., & Frazier, G. L., 1982, 'A model of strategy mix choice for planned social change', *J Market* 46:15–26.

Siegel, M., & Doner, L., 1998, *Marketing Public Health: Strategies to Promote Social Change*, Aspen Publishers, Gaithersburg, Md.

Sirgy, M. J., Morris, M., & Samli, A. C., 1985, 'The question of value in social marketing: use of a quality-of-life theory to achieve long-term satisfaction', *American Journal of Economics and Sociology* 44:215–28.

Wallack, L., Dorfman, L., Jernigan, D., & Themba, M., 1993, *Media Advocacy and Public Health: Power for Prevention*, Sage Publications, Newbury Park, Calif.

Walsh, D. C., Rudd, R. E., Moeykens, B. A., & Moloney, T. W., 1993, 'Social marketing for public health', *Health Affairs* 12:104–19.

Young, E., 1989, 'Social marketing in the information era', paper presented to the American Marketing Association Conference, Social Marketing for the 1990s, Ottawa.

Chapter 6
Focus on populations II: community approaches

Summary of main points

- The underlying purpose of community approaches in health promotion is to empower individuals and communities to gain control over the determinants of their own health.
- Capacity building is a means of empowering individuals, organisations and communities to do so.
- Partnerships are a key component of any successful health promotion program.
- Community organisation is a process of introducing positive changes for health in a community by involving that community in achieving largely predetermined goals.
- Community development involves the community in defining the agenda and changing itself with limited guidance and minimal intervention from outside.
- Without community participation, long-term health gains in populations are unlikely to be achieved.

The role of community processes

The subject of our first focus on populations, the mass media, are frequently used in health promotion as an 'umbrella' to set community agendas, promote awareness and increase knowledge on health issues while other health promotion processes occur. However, mass media programs, if used on their own, are not necessarily a magic bullet solution for achieving better health among populations.

Mass media methods in health promotion are seen by some as an imposition on a community by experts—sometimes from outside that community—with supposedly greater knowledge of what is good for that community. The questions this raises for public policy in a democratic society are obvious. Externally imposed mass media programs have also attracted the criticism that they do not address the underlying social and economic causes of health problems. They can also neglect the needs and idiosyncrasies of local communities.

Increasing focus on communities

Thompson and Kinne note the increasing focus on 'community' in health promotion, which they claim is due—at least in part—to 'a growing recognition that behaviour is greatly influenced by the environment in which people live. Proponents of community approaches to behavioural change recognise that local values, norms and behaviour patterns have a significant effect on shaping an individual's attitudes and behaviours' (Thompson & Kinne 1990).

It is too easy for health promotion practitioners to think they instinctively know what people need or what kind of program would be most suitable for any particular population group. The appropriate approach should be awareness of, and responsiveness to, the needs of the communities being served.

Many contemporary health promotion programs are targeted towards communities where health and social inequities are prevalent. These communities need to gain control of the determinants of their own health for their health status to improve. However, it is these same communities where individuals are often the most powerless. Therefore the health promotion practitioner needs to begin with an understanding of the role that empowerment plays in health and to possess skills in building empowerment among individuals and communities.

Empowerment is defined as 'access to, and control over, valued resources' (Katz 1984). This definition emphasises the establishment of an equitable distribution of resources to enable those presently disenfranchised and oppressed to experience a fair share of the power.

The Ottawa Charter for Health Promotion (WHO 1986) lists five principles for global health promotion action (see chapter 10). One of these is to strengthen community action to achieve better health. The Charter states: 'Health promotion works through concrete and effective community action in setting priorities, making decisions, planning strategies and implementing them to achieve better health. At the heart of this process is the empowerment of communities, their ownership and control of their own endeavours and destinies.' (WHO 1986)

Powerlessness, or lack of control over destiny, has emerged as a broad-based risk factor for disease (as discussed in chapter 1). Empowerment, although more difficult to evaluate, is also an important promoter of health. Wallerstein (1992) for example notes:

> Empowerment education ... involves people in group efforts to identify their problems, to critically assess social and historical roots of problems, to envision a healthier society, and to develop strategies to overcome obstacles in achieving their goals. Through community participation, people develop new beliefs in their ability to influence their personal and social spheres.

Community empowerment embodies an interactive process of change in which institutions and communities become transformed, as the people who participate in changing them become transformed. Rather than pitting individuals against community and overall societal needs, the community empowerment process focuses on both individual and community change (Wallerstein & Bernstein 1994).

Evaluation of community empowerment programs has presented challenges for program evaluators owing to the lack of standardised measures and the problem of finding appropriate indicators of program success. Nevertheless several published case studies provide reason for optimism in terms of progress in developing such measures (Eng & Parker 1994; Travers 1997).

The importance of community empowerment for health is borne out by studies over the years showing that programs emphasising individual preventive actions do not redress inequalities in health. In general, these studies have ascribed inequalities to the broad area of socioeconomic status (Cantor & Slater 1995; Smith, Taylor & Coates 1996; James et al. 1997) or more specifically to 'poverty' (Bolton et al. 1988). A closer analysis of the data (Syme 2003; Marmot 1994, 1999) reveals that the higher rates of morbidity and mortality in lower social classes cannot be attributed simply to lack of income. Other, less tangible factors associated with class— such as social support, the quality of the social and physical environment and the number of social stressors—need to be considered. It is unlikely that programs targeting individual risk factors alone will affect these deeper socioeconomic factors. Furthermore, as Travers (1997) cautions, in such situations, top-down health promotion strategies, such as dissemination of written information, 'may increase the differential between the advantaged and the disadvantaged by increasing the availability of resources—in this example, information—usable only by those already predisposed to healthy living with literacy skills and income sufficient to enable action on recommendations'.

To cope with this deficiency, strategies addressing change in communities from within have been developed. These include processes that have been called 'community organisation' and 'community development' but are often considered under the broad title of 'community approaches' (Bracht 1998). However, before undertaking these processes the health promotion practitioner needs to assess the capacity of the community and its various subgroups to address its health needs and support these changes where appropriate by strengthening this capacity.

The necessary elements for social change

Changes in health often require a social movement. Social movements in turn occur when a number of elements come together. These include a number of factors discussed by different writers (Kersh & Morone 2002; Brownell 2004) and modified for presentation here:

1. **An acknowledged crisis**. Little attention is paid to health issues until they morph into an obvious crisis, and particularly one that is felt personally.
2. **A critical mass of scientific evidence**. Vested interests will continue to complain about lack of evidence until it becomes overwhelming. At least 50 000 papers on the dangers of smoking had been published before cigarette manufacturers stopped being proactive about smoking.
3. **The obvious presence of victims**. Whether real or perceived, the injustice felt when victims are seen to be suffering is crucial to the mobilisation of opposition forces.
4. **A tug at the heart strings**. According to Brownell (2004): 'If there is any possibility for major social action and policy change, scientists cannot enforce it and health leaders cannot mandate it. The public must demand it.' Emotional involvement is the key to this happening. Emotions are most strongly aroused when children are seen to be victims.
5. **Strong political leadership**. Only when strong politicians are prepared to resist industry influence can a significant move be made towards social action. Whether this leads or follows other changes, however, varies according to circumstance.
6. **A balanced perspective**. Although vested interests can often be seen as total 'villains', most of them include ordinary people caught up in trying to make a living. Opposition groups should be rewarded and encouraged when positive actions are taken, as well as criticised when their actions are negative.

Capacity building

'Capacity building' is a process of facilitating people and communities to manage their own health. According to Hawe et al. (2001): 'Capacity building has been defined as being (at least) three activities: (1) building infrastructure to deliver health promotion programs; (2) building partnerships and organisational environments so that programs are sustained—and health gains are sustained; and (3) building problem-solving capability.'

Hawe et al. (2001) propose that capacity building can occur at five levels: one to one, in groups, in organisations, across organisations and across communities. Capacity building not only assists communities to help themselves to scarce resources but also empowers individuals (Eade 1997). This is based on the notion, expressed earlier, that much ill-health stems from social inequality, a sense of helplessness and discrimination or inability to access basic resources. According to Arole et al. (2004): 'Through the processes of information training, and imparting medical, economic, and social skills, individuals and communities gain in self-esteem and self-confidence, and come to realise that they have the capacity within themselves to determine their own lives.'

Principles for capacity building

Arole et al. (2004) list five key principles for capacity building. In summary, these are:

1. Community members must be involved in planning, implementing and evaluating programs. The most vulnerable must also be involved in all elements of a program. Community capacity building is about working in partnership and supporting community decision making.
2. Improving community capacity increases health by empowering communities to address underlying causes of ill health, such as lack of adequate nutrition, safe drinking water and clean environment.
3. Increased community capacity occurs through opportunities for increased networking and information exchange. Information sharing enhances community knowledge and methods of working together and allows community gaps to be identified and addressed.
4. Skill and knowledge transfer that supports capacity building is enhanced by relationships of mutual respect between the practitioner or program and the individual or community. One must respect the inherent capacity within all people and recognise that knowledge transfer is a two-way process.
5. Skills are best learned in practice, as distinct from the communication of a skill in an abstract conceptual way. Practice should be in the context of needs assessment, analysis of a situation, planning of a program, and implementation of activities.

Hawe et al. (2001) have developed a 'capacity building checklist' from which objective scores of capacity can be determined within communities and gaps identified for further action. For a fuller understanding of capacity building and this checklist, readers are referred to the publication.

Forming partnerships

Health promotion, perhaps more so than any other health discipline, cannot function in a vacuum. Interdisciplinary partnerships are needed at several different levels. Potential partners will be determined by the type of project in question. However, these can include government departments, local government bodies, relevant non-government organisations (e.g. Heart Foundation, diabetes associations, asthma groups, statistical collection groups, research bodies, private sector organisations), community groups and academic and educational institutions. Although the selection of these often seems obvious, a different perspective might need to be taken according to the diversity of the program. Reference materials are available for assisting health promotion practitioners to develop partnerships internationally (Pinet 2003), at the state level (Padget et al. 2004), or for specific issues, such as heart disease (Nchiinda 2003). Collaborative partnerships are a key component of community organisation and development processes.

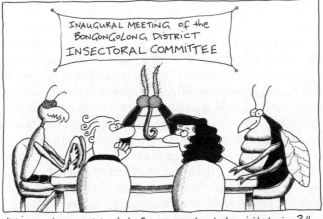

"Did you do a spellcheck before you sent out the invitations?"

Community organisation and community development

Both community organisation and community development have a considerable intellectual history outside the public health area, particularly within social work, sociology, community welfare and community psychology. Where community organisation ends and community development begins is often a grey area. The essential difference between the two, however, is the relative proportion of decision making and control invested in the community. In community development, this is greater than in community organisation.

Community organisation

Rothman (1968) defined three models of community organisation practice that remain valid today. These are social planning, social action and locality development.

Social planning emphasises a technical process of problem solving with regard to substantive social problems such as delinquency, housing and mental health. It is an approach that attempts to solve community problems rationally, within existing power structures. In this approach, community participation

Stages of social change

First they ignore you. Then they laugh at you. Then they fight you. Then you win.

Mahatma Gandhi

varies from a great deal to a little, depending on the nature of the situation. The approach presupposes a level of technical knowledge and skills among planners who, it is assumed, can skilfully guide complex change processes.

Social action is an activist approach that attempts to shift power structures in a community through various methods of coercion. It presupposes a generally disadvantaged or oppressed segment of the population that needs to be organised—perhaps in alliance with others—in order to make demands on the larger community for increased resources or treatment more in accordance with social justice. Examples are civil and worker rights, cause organisations and social movements, where combinations of the organisational and developmental roles exist.

Locality development aims to develop the potential of a community through self-help techniques and programs, within the constraints of the power structure. It rests on the assumption that community change can be pursued optimally through broad participation of a wide spectrum of people in goal determination and action at the local community level. Locality development is characterised by discussion and communication among a wide variety of different individuals, groups and factions, with the aim of achieving consensus. This model most closely approaches that of community develop-ment. Examples include neighbourhood work programs and community work in adult education.

In reality, health promotion practitioners need to draw on some combination of Rothman's three community organisation models. In some circumstances, the health issue might be significant enough to instigate a social movement for change.

The community organisation approach to health promotion has been most apparent in large-scale community projects such as in North Karelia, Finland (McAlister 1981), Stanford, California (Maccoby & Solomon 1981), Pawtucket, Rhode Island (Lasater, Carleton & LeFebvre 1988), the North Coast of New South Wales (Egger et al. 1983) and Wales (Nutbeam & Catford 1987). A review of community organisation programs for the prevention of cardiovascular diseases has also been undertaken by Mittelmark et al. (1993).

These large-scale public health programs have been comprehensive; that is, they have utilised a variety of different methods to achieve changes in individual behaviour and in community systems and structures. An acceptance of the multifactorial nature of behaviour and environmental change has resulted in an eclectic framework that draws on a variety of different theoretical models.

Case study 6.1

Injury prevention in Indigenous communities

Injury-related harm is a major cause of morbidity in Indigenous Australian communities. Hence replicable approaches to reducing injury are of considerable value to the health system as well as to Indigenous health and wellbeing.

A combination of a public health approach and community-owned and directed partnership processes have been used in an Indigenous community in Queensland. Outcome measures used were changes in the monthly incidence of injuries being reported over a two-year period.

Reported injuries decreased by a third in the community in the time of the trial, and statistical techniques showed that there was a 62 per cent probability that the shift in injury rates was associated with the introduction of the program. The principle of community management and ownership of the program supports the fact that that this is a key component of community-based programs.

Shannon et al. 2001

Whereas most of the large public health programs above have been initiated by a central health authority or agency—making them closest to social planning of the three community organisation models in Rothman's typology—it can be seen that information dissemination, behaviour change and maintenance of that change relies heavily on the involvement of community groups and organisations, which could provide a vehicle for locality or community development.

The activities of community organisation in these programs have included training of community members so that they can contribute to creating a supportive environment for those making behavioural changes. The longer-term objective in targeting whole communities is to influence the climate of opinion on health issues in communities so that behavioural and structural changes can occur. Influence can occur directly by placing issues on the community agenda, and by creating interest and controversy through exposure to media messages and events. Influence can also occur indirectly by reaching the informal communication networks or channels that exist in peer groups, families and institutions.

Methods of community organisation

Methods in community organisation vary widely, but basically involve the following actions:

- *Determining the health needs of the community in respect of quantifiable or qualifiable factors.* These could be related directly

Case study 6.2

The Stay On Your Feet program

In developed countries, falls are the major cause of unintentional injury and death among people 65 years and older, with approximately 30 per cent of the older adult population experiencing a fall each year. As a result of epidemiological work showing a high level of senior Australians and hospital admissions for falls in the region, Stay On Your Feet (SOYF), a community-based falls prevention program on the North Coast of New South Wales, was aimed at older people. Specific strategies included awareness raising through the electronic and print media and through other means, including the distribution of 24 000 informational books; community education, including the provision of affordable regular gentle exercise classes throughout the region; strategies targeting the urban environment in conjunction with local government and targeting the household environment through community health services; and a general practice strategy. Evaluation has shown a steady decline in falls and hospital admissions in the target population for up to eight years after the initiation of the project, which translated into a significant cost benefit.

Beard 2004

to health and determined from epidemiological statistics, or related indirectly, such as from community leaders' suggestions about the need for halfway houses. Methods include survey materials from the research literature, *ad hoc* surveys carried out by local government and other institutions, and formal and informal surveys with influential community members.

- *Involving the community in planning.* The main vehicle of community involvement in community organisation has typically been the community or interest group meeting, although the advent of modern two-way media has meant that radio and email can also be used, particularly in remote areas. Both are aided by the processes of publicity media referred to in chapter 5, as well as by direct invitation through interest groups. The latter is a more efficient technique because it has elements of personalisation. The organisation and running of planning functions should be carried out in as democratic a fashion as possible, although, in community organisation (compared with community development), the agenda is set and the meeting process must continually readdress that agenda. If necessary, changes could be facilitated in the task process so that community development takes over, but this should still address the objectives laid down in the community organisation brief.

- *Facilitating action.* The process of organisation and planning should have, as its outcome, some form of action. It can include further mobilisation of resources, development of programs, involvement in individual or group activities and social action where necessary. Action, and the outcome of such action, should be the cornerstone of the community organisation process, informing the health promotion practitioner of the success of their intervention.
- *Changing health outcomes.* In the process of social and community organisation, it is often easy to overlook the original intent; that is, to improve the health status of the individual and the community in which such organisation is taking place. This could require quantitative follow-up measures (e.g. risk factor assessments) or qualitative assessments of quality of life. However, subjective assessments of value of any program tend to be tainted with personal biases (only positive responders respond) and, although it might be tempting to ascribe negative or zero effects to independent variables, the health professional should be resilient enough to prosper from accurate feedback.

Case study 6.3

Using creative outcome measures— 'Bread: It's a Great Way to Go'

Three villages on the Mid North Coast of New South Wales with a high proportion of retirees were chosen to test the effects of increased bread consumption on constipation. Although there was no health educational material in the program that mentioned laxative use, sales of laxatives through local chemists was used as a proxy measure of constipation and hence a potential outcome measure. Social marketing, advice from general practitioners and community organisation was used in village A; village B used only advice from local GPs; and village C acted as a control with no intervention carried out. After six months, bread sales had increased by 50 per cent and laxative sales had decreased by more than 60 per cent in village A, compared with both villages B and C, suggesting that an increase in the promotion of fibre (through bread) could have an indirect effect on constipation and hence laxative sales.

Egger et al. 1991

Appropriate situations for community organisation

Community organisation in some form is appropriate to most health promotion situations (Wakefield & Wilson 1985). Community organisation could link with individual, group and mass media methods where a strategy mix will require concurrent intervention at individual, group and population levels. In the case of the use of mass media, it is clearly indicated (Flay 1987; Redman, Spencer & Sanson-Fisher 1990) that media programs alone are not as effective as programs in which media exposure is accompanied by community organisation.

The mass media alone will not be effective unless organisational, economic and environmental changes enable, and interpersonal communications reinforce, the behavioural change objectives.

Case study 6.4

The success of learning from failures

Successes in health promotion are nice to report, yet learning also occurs from failures. Community public health approaches have been successful in some areas, particularly smoking, injury prevention and so on, as discussed in other parts of this book. To date, however, there has been little success in dealing with one of the world's newest epidemics: obesity. In several attempts to reduce obesity at the population level through community approaches, Professor Robert Jeffery, from the University of Massachusetts, admits to limited, if any, success (Jeffery 2001). The implication might be that population-level approaches will not work where risk factors (over-eating and inactivity) are enticing. However, another explanation could be that without attention to upstream factors influencing obesity, such as the 'obesogenic' environment and vector factors (high energy-dense, processed foods and abundant energy-saving technology), population approaches could be expected to have only limited effect. This would imply, as the epidemiological triad discussed in chapter 1 suggests, that all, and not just any, corners of the triad need to be addressed before any major influence on an epidemic can occur.

Community development

Community development is the process of involving communities from the ground up in their own decision making about factors related to health (Allen 1997). It concerns working with people and communities to develop their strength and confidence over an extended time period, as well as addressing immediate and pressing problems (Baum 1989).

Until 1950, the community development process was generally characterised by government intervention with a view to teaching 'backward people' better techniques for managing their land and their health, or to overcome 'the inadequacies of colonial services in the fields of education, health and welfare' (Dixon 1989). Whereas self-help was stressed within the process, self-determination was not on the agenda, and community development, it appears, was wittingly and unwittingly used to create dependency on the sponsoring body rather than independence from this body. Dixon (1989) reviews more recent developments:

> In public-policy terms, community development has, since the sixties, been a popular means of fostering participation in local-area service delivery, of obtaining the views and compliance of local leaders through consultation, and of encouraging self-help, volunteerism and cost-saving decentralisation. More recently, the securing of a sense of 'we-feeling' to counteract the problems of powerlessness and anomie, and to propel groups to collective action has been highlighted as valuable in the fields of local economic development, community mental health, adult education and social welfare.

Shabecoff and Brophy (2001) define 'community development' as 'the economic, physical and social revitalisation of a community; led by the people who live in that community'. In this sense 'community developers do things with, not to or for, the community'.

Fiske et al. (1989) claim that community development in health is

> a challenge to the individualist focus of conventional sick care. Sick-care services can be delivered in ways which harness and build community support or they can isolate the patient and the family from the various communities of which they are a part and, in doing so, deny the patient those supports and weaken those communities.

Case study 6.5

A community activity program for women

'Concord, a great place to be active' is the name of a health promotion program established in a Sydney suburb, aimed at increasing activity levels of 20–50-year-old women. The program used a combination of strategies, including partnership arrangements with the local council, capacity building, social marketing and community organisation. Environmental changes also made activity more feasible in the area. Following the intervention there was a statistically significant (6.4 per cent) reduction in the proportion of sedentary women in the area after two years of the program. There were also a number of positive changes made in the local council's capacity to promote physical activity. As inactivity is a major cause of health problems, programs such as this, which increase activity levels by small amounts in large populations, could be expected to have a significant influence over time.

Li Ming et al. 2004

Lin (1989) has observed that, whereas community development in health promotion had previously been translated as 'the health promotion officer will do whatever the community wants him/her to do', there is now sufficient practice to develop a more rigorous approach to community development in health.

In health promotion, the community development perspective emphasises the importance of conceiving health promotion programs through a negotiated partnership with the communities whose cooperation and participation the health promotion practitioner seeks. A precondition for negotiations is an acceptance by the practitioner that the proposed program design might not be regarded as suitable by the communities to whom it is offered, or that management control might have to be shared.

Applying community development

The nature of community development processes implies that they will be more effective among communities and sections of communities who are disempowered, where continuing inequalities exist with respect to health experience across class, gender, race and ethnicity, and where these groups are without the economic and social means to make decisions about their own lives (Jackson et al. 1989). In Green and McAlister's terms, these are the 'hardest to reach' and are most likely to have the poorest health status. They are people who are

> typically disadvantaged in economic or status terms, they are socially more isolated or alienated, and they tend to be suspicious of organisations, including government agencies, purporting to help them. Their use of media is more exclusively for entertainment and their membership in organisations or coalitions is sporadic and limited to comparison with the early adopters. Reaching these people and organisations requires more expensive and labour-intensive forms of community organisation, communication and outreach. The payoff is often greater because of their high risk, but the cost per unit of service effectively delivered is necessarily higher. (Green & McAlister 1984)

The community development approach then is most appropriate for, and can claim some successes in, lower socioeconomic and disadvantaged groups, such as in developing countries (Oakley 1989), among lower-income groups (El-Askari et al. 1998) and with Indigenous people (Coperman 1988). However, in some areas of concern, such as drug and alcohol abuse, community development approaches have been influential among all income groups (Reilly & Hommel 1988). These approaches have involved local schools, clubs, local governments and concerned citizens.

The role of the health promotion practitioner in the community development process is as a facilitator of action; to be as unobtrusive as possible, but to ensure that things happen. This role is not always an easy one and ethical dilemmas could arise for community organisers and developers—including health promotion practitioners—as they attempt to reconcile their mandate from both their employers and their communities, particularly if there are conflicting agendas (Minkler 1978). These realities are the reason community developers are not always popular with everyone and are sometimes regarded as 'ratbags'. However, Baum (1990) reminds us that the first Medical Officers of Health appointed under the UK's Health of Towns movement in the nineteenth century could have been regarded as 'troublemakers' for health. In the context of the charter of the 'new public health', Baum suggests: 'we must be prepared to be troublemakers for health—to rock the boat, to challenge the status quo and, perhaps most importantly, to question our own way of working and ensure our practice matches the rhetoric' (Baum 1990).

In summary, then, community development in health should include the following elements:

- a thorough knowledge of the health and health-associated problems of the area involved
- a thorough knowledge of the community itself: population, class, age structure, resources, power groups, knowledge of the normal processes of community action
- identification of leaders and influential people in the appropriate areas in the community, both elected and natural
- identification of natural neighbourhoods (see Kowachi & Berkman 2003)
- any opinion surveys that might have been conducted in the community
- natural organisation of concerned groups and coalitions to consider identified problems
- emergence of representative planning groups to establish goals and plans for action
- development of neighbourhood committees
- training of volunteers if needed
- consistent feedback
- utilisation of the available media, and
- maintained momentum.

Summary of community organisation and community development

Community organisation and community development differ in the degree of control and centralisation over program management that is held within the community itself. Community organisation principles are fundamental to most health promotion programs—particularly those in which media are involved and which have a set agenda. Community development is most appropriate in lower socioeconomic and disadvantaged settings with hard-to-reach individuals. Both systems have elements that are vital to the process of health promotion.

Career opportunities in health promotion

Health promotion work involving capacity building, community development and community organisation is usually part of a generalist health promotion practitioner's role. Work in this field as a health promotion speciality is available in developing countries through aid organisations and professional consulting firms as well as with the World Health Organization. Local government and community-based organisations, such as youth and seniors organisations, require workers with these skills. Health departments also employ health promotion officers specialising in community development and community organisation processes, particularly for rural and remote areas and in Indigenous communities. Community welfare and social workers are involved in capacity building through local and non-government organisations. Capacity building skills are also sought after in private sector work for applications in coalition building, environmental and community planning and organisational development. For more detailed information on careers in community development see Shabecoff and Brophy (2001).

References

Allen, C. F., 1997, 'Community development for health and identity politics', *Ethnic Health* 2(3):229–42.

Arole, R., Fuller, B., & Deutschmann, P., 2004, 'Improving community capacity', in Moodie, R., & Hulme, A. (eds), *Hands-on Health Promotion*, IP Communications, Melbourne, Vic.

Baum, F., 1989, 'Editorial: community development and the new public health in Australia and New Zealand', *Comm Health Stud*. 13(1):1–3.

—— 1990, 'Troublemakers for health?', *In Touch* 7(1):5–6.

Beard, J., 2004, 'Long-term follow-up and economic evaluation of a falls prevention program: population strategies are successful, sustained and cost effective', unpublished report, Department of Rural Health, Southern Cross University, Lismore, NSW.

Bolton, S., Broadhead, P., Budd, J., Duckett, S. & Gifford, S., 1988, 'Who "needs" community health? Planning for equity in the distribution of scarce resources', *Comm Health Stud* 12(3):256–63.

Bracht, N. F., 1998, *Health Promotion at the Community Level: New Advances* (2nd edn), Sage Publications, Thousand Oaks, Calif.

Brownell, K. D., 2004, *Food Fight*, Contemporary Books, New York.

Cantor, C. H., & Slater, P. J., 1995, 'Socioeconomic indices and suicide rate in Queensland', *Aust J Pub Health* 19(3):417–20.

Coperman, R. C., 1988, 'Assessment of Aboriginal health services', *Comm Health Stud* 12(3):251–60.

Dixon, J., 1989, 'The limits and potential of community development for personal and social change', *Comm Health Stud* 13(1):82–92.

Eade, D., 1997, *Capacity Building: An Approach to People-centred Development*, Oxfam, London.

Egger, G., Fitzgerald, W., Frape, G., Monaem, A., Rubinstein, P., Tyler, C., & Mackay, B., 1983, 'Results of a large-scale media anti-smoking campaign in Australia: The North Coast Healthy Lifestyle Programme', *Brit Med J* 287:1125–87.

Egger, G., Wolfenden, K., Pares, J., Mowbray, G., 1991, '"Bread: it's a great way to go": increasing bread consumption decreases laxative sales in an elderly community', *Med J Aust*, 155(11–12):820–1.

El-Askari, G., Freestone, J., Irizarry, C., Kraut, K. L., Mashiyama, S. T., Morgan, M. A., & Walton, S., 1998, 'The Healthy Neighbourhoods Project: a local health department's role in catalyzing community development', *Health Ed & Behav* 25(2):146–59.

Elder, R. W., Shultz, R. A., Sleet, D. A., Nichols, J. L., Thompson, R. S., & Warda, R., 2004, 'Effectiveness of mass media campaigns for reducing drinking and driving and alcohol involved crashes', *Amer J Prev Med*, 27(1):57–65.

Eng, E., & Parker, E., 1994, 'Measuring community competence in the Mississippi Delta: the interface between program evaluation and empowerment', *Health Ed Quart* 21(2):199–220.

Fiske, G., Hill, A., Krouskos, D., Legge, D., & Stagoll, O., 1989, 'The Community Development in Health Project', *Comm Health Stud* 13(1):93–9.

Flay, B. R., 1987, 'Mass media and smoking cessation: a critical review', *Am J Pub Health* 77(2):153–60.

Green, L. W., & McAlister, A. L., 1984, 'Macro-intervention to support health behaviour: some theoretical perspectives and practical reflections', *Health Ed Quart* 11(3):332–9.

Hawe, P., King, L., Noort, M., Jornens, C., & Lloyd, B., 2001, *Indicators to Help with Capacity Building in Health Promotion*, Australian Centre for Health Promotion, NSW Health, Sydney.

Jackson, T., Mitchell, S., & Wright, M., 1989, 'The community development continuum', *Community Health Studies* 13(1):66–73.

James, W. P. T., Nelson, M., Ralph, A., & Leather, S., 1997, 'The contribution of nutrition to inequalities in health', *Brit Med J* 314:1545–9.

Jeffery, R. W., 2001, 'Public health strategies for obesity treatment and prevention', *Am J Health Behav* 25(3):252–9.

Katz, R., 1984, *Empowerment and Synergy: Expanding the Community's Healing Resources*, *Studies in Empowerment* (series), Haworth Press, New York.

Kersh, R., & Morone, J., 2002, 'How the personal becomes political: prohibitions, public health and obesity', *Stud Am Pol Devel* 16:162–75.

Kowachi, I., & Berkman, L. F. (eds), 2003, *Neighbourhoods and Health*, Oxford University Press, Oxford.

Lasater, T. M., Carleton, R. A., & LeFebvre, R. C., 1988, 'The Pawtucket Heart Health Programme: utilizing community resources for primary prevention', *Rhode Island Med J* 71:63–7.

Li Ming, W., Thomas, M., Jones, H., Orr, N., Moreton, R., King, L., Hawe, P., Bindon, J., Humphries, J., Schicht, K., Corne, A., & Bauman, A., 2002, 'Promoting physical activity in women: evaluation of a two-year community-based intervention in Sydney, Australia', *Health Prom Int* 17(2):127–37.

Lin, V., 1989, 'Education, prevention and social realities', paper presented at the Fourth National Drug Educators' Workshop, Adelaide, SA.

Maccoby, N., & Solomon, D. S., 1981, 'The Stanford Community Studies in Heart Disease Prevention', in Rice, R. E., & Paisley, W. J. (eds), *Public Communication Campaigns*, Sage Publications, Beverly Hills, Calif.

Marmot, M. G., 1994, 'Social differentials in health within and between populations', *Daedalus* 4:197–216.

—— 1999, *Social Determinants of Health*, Oxford University Press, Oxford.

McAlister, A., 1981, 'Anti-smoking campaigns: progress in developing effective communications', in Rice, R. E., & Paisley, W. J. (eds), *Public Communication Campaigns*. Sage Publications, Beverly Hills, Calif.

Minkler, M., 1978, 'Ethical issues in community organization', *Health Ed Monog* Summer:198–210.

Mittelmark, M. B., Hunt, M. K., Heath, G. W., & Schmidt, T. L., 1993, 'Realistic outcomes: lessons from community-based research and demonstration programs for the prevention of cardiovascular diseases', *J Pub Health Pol* 14:437–62.

Nchiinda, T. C., 2003, 'Research capacity development for CVD prevention: the role of partnerships', *Ethn Dis* 13(2 Suppl 2):540–4.

Nutbeam, D., & Catford, J., 1987, 'The Welsh Heart Program evaluation strategy: progress, plans and possibilities', *Health Prom* 2(1):5–18.

Oakley, P., 1989, *Community Involvement in Health Development: An Examination of the Critical Issues*, World Health Organization, Geneva.

Padget, S. M., Bekemeier, B., & Berkowitz, B., 2004, 'Collaborative partnerships at the state level: promoting systems changes in public health infrastructure', *J Pub Health Manag Pract* 10(3):251–7.

Pinet, G., 2003, 'Global partnerships: a key challenge and opportunity for implementation of international health law', *Med Law* 22(4):561–77.

Redman, S., Spencer, E., & Sanson-Fisher, R., 1990, 'The role of the mass media in changing health related behaviour: a critical appraisal of two models', *Health Prom Int* 5(1):85–101.

Reilly, C., & Hommel, P., 1988, *Strategies for the Prevention of Drug and Alcohol Problems*, Directorate of the Drug Offensive, New South Wales Department of Health, Sydney.

Rothman, J., 1968, 'Three models of community organisation practice', National Conference on Social Welfare, Social Work Practice, Columbia University Press, New York.

Shabecoff, A., & Brophy C., 2001, *A Guide to Careers in Community Development*. Island Press, New York.

Shannon, C., Canuto, C., Young, E., Craig, D., Schluter, P., Kenny, G., & McClure, R., 2001, 'Injury prevention in Indigenous communities: results of a two-year community development project', *Health Prom J Aust* 12(3):233–7.

Smith, D., Taylor, R., & Coates, M., 1996, 'Socioeconomic differentials in cancer incidence and mortality in urban New South Wales 1987–91', *Aust & NZ J Pub Health* 20(2):129–37.

Syme, L. S., 2003, 'Social determinants of health: the community as empowered partner', paper presented to the Communities in Control Conference (convened by Community and Catholic Social Services), Melbourne, Vic.

Thompson, B., & Kinne, S., 1990, 'Social change theory: applications to community health', in Bracht, N. (ed.), *Health Promotion at the Community Level*, Sage Pubications, Newbury Park, Calif., pp. 45–65.

Travers, K., 1997, 'Reducing inequities through participatory research and community empowerment', *Health Ed & Behav* 24(3):344–56.

Wakefield, M. A., & Wilson, D. A., 1985, 'Community organisation for health promotion', *Comm Health Stud* 10(4):444–50.

Wallerstein, N., 1992, 'Powerlessness, empowerment and health: implications for health promotion programs', *Am J Health Prom* 6(3):197–205.

Wallerstein, N., & Bernstein, E., 1994, 'Introduction to community empowerment, participatory education and health', *Health Educ Quart* 21(2):141–8.

WHO (World Health Organization), 1986, *Ottawa Charter for Health Promotion*, International Conference on Health Promotion, Ottawa.

Chapter 7
Focus on populations III: environmental approaches

Summary of main points

- By making the healthy choice an easier choice (and sometimes the only choice) environmental approaches can be more effective than trying to change behaviour to achieve better health.
- Environments can be thought of as physical, economic, sociocultural or political.
- Environmental interventions include policy, regulation and legislation, technological changes, organisational interventions and the use of incentives and disincentives.
- Technological change, such as the use of sun creams for skin cancer, represents a positive advance for health promotion.
- The ANGELO process is one way of diagnosing unhealthy environments
- Economic and political considerations weigh heavily on environmental issues.
- Without economic and environmental attention, health promotion can be like 'cooking dinner while the house is burning'.

The value of passive change

The strategies and methods dealt with so far in this book involve direct interventions with individuals, groups or whole populations, often focusing on intrapersonal and interpersonal factors. Another, more indirect means of influencing a population's health is by passively changing environments that encourage ill-health, with interventions from direct manipulation of the environment, to the development of healthy public policy, ranging from the introduction of regulations and legislation, and organisational and other settings-based adaptations, to the application of incentives and disincentives. Systems-based environmental interventions can add to the often modest influence of other health promotion programs (Kickbush 1997; Harris & Wills 1997).

The importance of creating supportive environments achieved formal recognition with the Ottawa Charter in 1986. Since then, more sophisticated environmental models have been developed for dealing with a variety of contemporary health issues (Sallis & Owen 1996; Nutbeam 1997; Egger & Swinburn 1997). Environments in this context should not be considered only as physical. They also include economic, political or sociocultural environments. In addition, there are micro-environments, or those in immediate proximity to the target population, sometimes considered as 'settings'; and macro-environments, or those encompassing industry, economic and employment groups and considered as 'sectors'.

As Steckler et al. (1995) have observed in the USA, the social, political and economic environment could encourage or reinforce health-damaging behaviour and might discourage people from even desiring to engage in healthy behaviour. For example advertisements for cigarettes and alcoholic drinks often create a social environment that makes smoking or drinking look like the road to success and popularity (Pierce et al. 1994; US Department of Health and Human Services 1994). The environment could also discourage people from engaging in health-enhancing actions—even when they want to do so—by providing obstacles like high prices, lack of availability and social stigma to such behaviour.

Health promoting policies can modify social, political and economic influences. For example to discourage smoking, especially among adolescents, health promotion advocates have successfully lobbied for increased taxes on tobacco products, especially to discourage the uptake of smoking (Bierer & Rigotti 1992). Environmental measures have the advantage of cost-effectiveness, influencing population groups that are often hard to reach and having a more lasting effect on behaviour change because they become incorporated into structures, systems, policies and sociocultural norms (Swinburn, Egger & Raza 1999).

The approaches that can be considered under the strategy of environmental adaptations are:

- modifications to the environment
- changes in public policy
- regulation and legislation
- technological interventions
- organisational interventions, and
- the use of incentives and disincentives.

Advocacy for change could also be considered in this category, but because it has been considered in relation to social marketing in chapter 5, it will not be discussed again here.

Case study 7.1

The subtle influence of the environment

Some novel Australian research shows how small subtle changes in the environment can mount to have a large long-term influence on health. A group of actors who play the part of soldiers, convicts and settlers at Old Sydney Town, a theme park north of Sydney in New South Wales, were asked to live in for a week and not use modern technology at all during that time while wearing special movement sensors to detect activity levels. Results were then compared with that of a group of sedentary urban office workers in modern-day Sydney. The average difference amounted to around 1000 kcals of energy per day, or the equivalent of walking approximately 16 km more in the early nineteenth century than in the early twenty-first century.

A theoretical postulation of changes in activity levels is shown in figure 7.1.

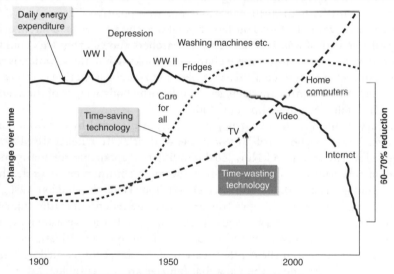

*Changes shown are hypothetical and not based on actual data

Figure 7.1: Postulated changes in physical activity levels over time with changes in technology (from Vogels et al. 2004)

This suggests that although activity levels in the general population would have been expected to increase during the Great Depression and both world wars, big decreases probably coincided with the introduction of time-saving technology (e.g. cars, refrigerators, washing machines and so on) after the 1950s. This was increased by the development of time-using technology (videos, electronic games, TV) and more recently by the significant effects of the Internet. Such declines show the power of the environment in affecting modern health, and are likely to have contributed significantly to the modern obesity epidemic.

Vogels et al. 2004

Modifying the environment

Behaviour of a long-standing nature—such as diet or exercise—is notoriously difficult to change. Changes to the physical environment, which are of positive benefit, can sometimes be made more easily. For example traffic accident research shows that the fatality rate from motor vehicles is significantly decreased on dual-lane highways compared with single lanes (Campkin 1990).

Another example is in the area of nutrition. It is now well accepted that a lowering of total fat in the diet is a vital aspect of improving the health of the population. However, because high-fat foods are readily available, tasty and cheap, it is difficult to influence behaviour in a positive direction. In New Zealand, a survey of fast-food outlets showed that the average fat content of hot chips (French fries) was 11.5 per cent. Researchers showed that this could be reduced by 1.5 per cent by simple changes in cooking practices, which would then result in an estimated decrease in per capita fat consumption of 0.5 kg per year and hence a significant decrease in unhealthy body weight of the average New Zealander (Morley-John et al. 2002).

Injury is another area that is particularly influenced by environmental change. Injury is the third-largest cause of death (after heart disease and cancers) in Australia and New Zealand, but is responsible for many more years of potential life lost because it is the most common cause of death in those younger than 40. US engineer Dr William Haddon (Haddon 1980) led a paradigm shift in thinking in this area when he redefined traffic injury in epidemiological terms and showed that the appropriate intervention for injury prevention is relatively easy and requires only simple modifications to the environment (although these modifications must be accompanied by a shift in community attitude to the view that injuries are preventable).

Successes in injury prevention through environmental modifications include:

- a 27 per cent decrease in rates of injury in the home resulting from involvement of local community groups in improving the home environment for better safety (Schelp 1987)
- reduction in injuries in children through the substitution of safety glass in windows in high-risk areas (Oliver & Lawson 1979)
- a 73 per cent reduction in swimming pool drownings in children through erection of proper barriers around home pools (Thompson & Rivara 2003), and

Case study 7.2

Changing ships for better health

The influence of subtle changes in the environment on health is exemplified by a US Navy study that compared surreptitious changes to a low fat diet in one US Navy ship with a second ship on which no such change occurred over a six-month deployment. Cooks on the test ship (ship A) were instructed on cooking to American Cardiology Society (ACS) guidelines. Exercise was also encouraged in the test ship, but shops and vending machines remained unchanged. Standard navy menus were unchanged on the control ship (ship B).

Results after six months (shown in the table below) suggest a major impact of a subtle change in ship A's environment.

	Ship A	Ship B
Mean weight change	−5.3 kg	+3.1 kg
Mean waist change	−4.8 cm	+3.6 cm
In those greater than 90 kg at start	74% lost weight 26% gained weight	26% lost weight 74% gained weight

Swinburn 2002

- a 50 per cent decrease in sports injuries in Sweden through the introduction of a prophylactic program including ankle taping, stretching, controlled rehabilitation, optimal equipment and selection of players (Eckstrand 1989).

The lesson from these examples is that if there are choices of strategy, a first priority should be to seek to alter the environment before tackling more difficult behavioural or social changes (Mock et al. 2004). A National Injury Surveillance Unit (NISU) was established as a federal initiative to monitor causes and changes of injuries throughout Australia. State health departments have now also taken on the role of injury prevention, and some states have bodies for reducing specific injuries, such as through motor vehicle accidents.

Healthy public policy

Policy change is another effective means of modifying unhealthy environments. One-off interventions can improve health for certain groups at particular times, but for sustained and comprehensive change for better health, environmental adaptations must become the subject of public policy.

Building healthy public policy is one of the five areas listed for action in the Ottawa Charter for Health Promotion (WHO 1986). This means that in all sections and at all levels of government (including local, regional and national levels), policy makers must be aware of and accept responsibility for the health consequences of their decisions. It also means that a range of measures, including some of those described in this chapter, should be used to effect and maintain positive action.

Industry policy changes required for control of obesity in children

Food sales and marketing have become a major concern in light of big increases in obesity in school-age children around the world. In a comprehensive analysis of approaches to deal with the problem, US obesity expert Dr Kelly Brownell has suggested:

> the time has come for the [food and soft drink] industry to determine that it will be a trustworthy public health ally by adopting the following practices: (1) suspend all food advertising and marketing campaigns directed at children; (2) remove sugar-sweetened soft drinks and snack foods from vending machines in schools; (3) end sponsorship of scholastic activities and professional nutrition organisations linked to product promotion; and (4) refrain from political contributions that might influence national nutritional policy. (Brownell 2004)

In a surprise move in Australia in 2004, a major soft drink manufacturing company announced that it will conform with at least the first three of Brownell's proposals (the fourth has not been discussed), leaving the way open for a new relationships between some industries and health.

In practice, policy decisions and strategies are most often expressed in legislation, which became a cornerstone of public health in its response in the nineteenth century to epidemics and unsanitary living conditions. A broader and newer application is the fostering of public participation and intersectoral cooperation wherever regulations and legislation are proposed that will affect health.

It is also necessary to recognise that a wide range of government agencies operating in areas of legislative responsibility beyond the traditional health sector also have important contributions to make in protecting and improving public health. This both widens and strengthens the role that legislation plays in this area. Transport, housing, employment, agriculture, fisheries, power and business can all exert influence in the health arena, particularly on social inequalities that lead to ill-health.

Case study 7.3

ANGELO: a diagnostic tool for identifying unhealthy environments

ANGELO, an ANalysis Grid for Environments Leading to Obesity, was developed initially to help communities diagnose aspects of their environment that could enhance or discourage obesity and identify potential interventions. The grid consists of four environmental types and two sizes (see text for a discussion of these) defining settings and sectors in a community.

The questions shown in table 7.1 are put to stakeholders to identify key obesogenic elements and these are then ranked according to local relevance, potential impact and changeability, to identify high priority areas for intervention.

Table 7.1: A grid for diagnosing environments

Environment type/size	Micro-environment (settings)		Macro-environment (sectors)	
	Food	Physical activity	Food	Physical activity
Physical	What is available?			
Economic	What are the financial factors?			
Policy	What are the rules?			
Sociocultural	What are the attitudes, beliefs, perceptions and values?			

The grid has been used with stakeholder groups in several Pacific Island communities to encourage community participation and focus actions for 'diabesity' prevention. After getting stakeholders to fill in the matrix by brainstorming environmental issues, the grid is then 'lifted' and choices ranked with consideration of possible solutions.

The ANGELO approach is a facilitatory tool, which enables community members to recognise causal issues that might otherwise be less clear. Examples from the Pacific include roaming dogs that stop islanders walking (physical environment), attitudes to women exercising in public and during pregnancy (sociocultural), cost and availability of low-fat fresh food (economic), and excessive TV watching among children (changes in family politics).

ANGELO is not meant to provide answers to environmental issues. These should come from the community itself. It does, however, provide an enlightened perspective and community involvement in ongoing interventions.

Swinburn, Egger & Raza 1999

Regulation and legislation

In some circumstances, legislation (by making the healthy choice the only choice), backed up by policing, is another effective way of influencing behaviour. For example the compulsory wearing of seatbelts and breathalyser control of drink-driving have resulted in a decrease in road traffic accidents in most areas where they have been introduced. These measures were effective only when they were made compulsory and only when police monitored compulsion. The significant difference in traffic accident injury rates between Australia and the USA has been attributed to the early introduction of compulsory seatbelt use and drink-driver restrictions in Australia. Differences in homicide rates between the two countries have similarly been put down to firearm enforcement laws in Australia (Sleet 1990).

Legislation and policing without compulsion might be acceptable to a particular segment of the population. Smoking is an example. To ban tobacco smoking formally would not be acceptable to many people because it would be seen as a denial of an individual's democratic right to smoke, and because of the effect a ban would have on black-market sales of cigarettes and associated criminal activities. However, gradual changes in community attitudes to smoking have resulted in greater acceptance of smoking legislation and voluntary changes, such as banning smoking from workplaces, theatres, public transport and aircraft, and provision of non-smoking sections in restaurants (Chapman et al. 1990). However, a considered analysis of improvements in smoking levels has shown that although improvements have been considerable, they could be much greater with more committed government support. Chapman (2004) for example explains that although just $176 million was spent on tobacco control in Australia from 1970 to 1998, the benefits accruing to government in the same period were $8.4 billion.

Introducing new legislation can be a long-term process. Because the health promotion practitioner often works in a restricted environment, the power of one person to influence legislative change is limited (although not impossible). Health promotion practitioners might need to utilise some of the strategies of community organisation suggested in chapter 6 to mobilise public demand and/or acceptance of new legislation.

Communities must also consider and debate the question of how much control should be vested in the state to legislate in matters that could be viewed as compromising democratic freedoms and the rights of free citizens. However, even where there is initial resistance, legislation that can demonstrate its benefits in protecting health can gain public acceptance after its introduction. For example, in 1990, the New South Wales Government introduced the Swimming Pools Act to ensure that all residential pools were isolated from living areas and neighbouring property by a childproof fence. The Act was the first of its kind in Australia and was in the precarious position of setting an example for other states to follow. The Act also faced considerable opposition from special interest groups. However, after it was introduced, a survey by Elkington, Carey and Fowler (1992) found that, among pool owners, 85 per cent indicated that they approved of compulsory isolation fencing and, even among pool owners who had yet to comply with the legislation, 70 per cent approved of the requirements.

At the micro-environmental level, regulation can include local rules, regulations and policies that can have profound effects on the behaviour of individuals and organisations. An example is policy within schools relating to food, which can influence options in school meals, vending machines and tuck shops (Nutbeam 1997). The home is another important micro setting in which family 'rules' about food purchase and consumption can alter the 'obesogenicity' of the home environment.

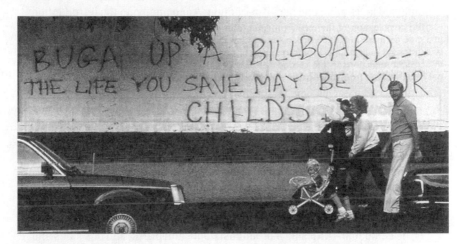

The work of BUGAUP (Billboard Utilising Graphitists Against Unhealthy Promotions) to change the health environment in the 1980s

Ordinance changes can occur at the local government level as a result of lobbying, deputations, letter writing from local constituents and community action. A now well-developed technique for instituting action at the government level is the circulation of prepared forms for constituents to sign, send or email to local MPs and authorities. Because a form removes two of the major barriers to individual action (i.e. time and effort), it can facilitate action. Lobby groups that have been effective in building momentum for legislative changes in health through consistent advocacy (and sometimes utilising social action—see chapter 6) include:

- Action on Smoking and Health (ASH)
- the non-smokers' rights movement
- Billboard Utilising Graffitists Against Unhealthy Promotions (BUGAUP)

- Consumers' Health Forum
- People Against Drink Driving (PADD)
- Mothers Against Drink Driving (MADD)
- Australian Consumers Association (ACA), and
- Australian Nutrition Foundation (ANF).

Case study 7.4

How will you go when you sit for the test ...?

The introduction of drinking restrictions on drivers in New South Wales in 1982, requiring a blood-alcohol level of under 0.05 per cent, is an example of one of the most effective health promotion strategies of recent times. It combined legislation and social marketing. Accompanying the introduction of the law was a strategically devised advertising campaign designed on the basis of qualitative research indicating that drivers would not be influenced by appeals to social responsibility or fear of personal injury but were concerned about the social embarrassment of being arrested.

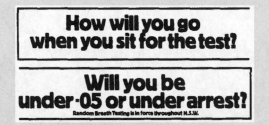

The campaign—utilising a broadcast jingle and press, and bus sides and bumper stickers—used the slogan: 'How will you go when you sit for the test? Will you be under .05 or under arrest?'

The combination of legislation and the media program (plus the publicity generated) resulted in a 40 per cent decrease in traffic accidents in New South Wales in the first year of operation. However, a lack of visibility of breath testing units and lack of knowledge of people who had been arrested led to a decline in accident reductions in the second year of operation. This resulted in police later carrying out breath testing from patrol cars, which were also more visible.

Bevins 1988

Technological interventions

Although changes in behaviour are a significant factor in disease epidemiology, technological advances should also be considered as a potential underlying cause. Hence it is Bill Gates, who could be accused of causing the increase in population levels of sedentariness at the turn of the century through the sophistication of effort-saving technology, perhaps as much as Ronald McDonald, or other fast-food purveyors. Technological interventions involve changes in preventive health brought about through improvements in medical and scientific technology. These include insecticides to reduce infection-carrying insects; immunisation; fluoridation of the water supply; motor vehicle safety engineering, such as airbags, seatbelts and median barriers; exercise machines; low-fat and energy-dense food technology; sun and skin creams—to name a few.

Technological interventions are generally the domain of the medical, engineering or environmental expert. However, implementation and acceptance of such developments is often left to the health promotion practitioner. The development of sunscreens to filter out the harmful effects of short-wave ultraviolet light, for example, has been a technological innovation with beneficial consequences for those exposed to sunlight. But health promotion interventions are necessary to inform those at risk about the use of such screens and to develop programs to counter social norms that inhibit the use of such innovations (McCarthy & Shaw 1989).

The range of industrial safety devices (such as safety goggles, hoods over circular saws, and the wearing of protective helmets and boots) has added considerably to industrial and occupational safety. The reduction of noise through engineering techniques has been a major factor in the reduction of loss of hearing owing to industrial and other noise.

The accelerating pace of technology shows no signs of slowing down as we begin the twenty-first century. This has provided mixed blessings for health; fast food and labour-saving home appliances being cases in point. However, it is the health promotion practitioner who might have the most crucial role to play in identifying technology that shows most promise for health gain and in building community support for its introduction and implementation. The use of exercise machines, active entertainment, such as dance machines in fun parlours, television and video games driven by exercise bicycles and activity sensors with devices for switching off electronics if enough movement is not carried out, are examples of the use of technology to deal with the problems that technology has created (Egger, Swinburn & Rossner 2002). This will undoubtedly become a growth area of the future.

Organisational interventions

A major problem for health promotion is reaching the population targeted for intervention in sufficient numbers for the costs involved. For this reason, specific settings exist that enable greater access to 'captive' groups. This can include the workplace, schools, churches and other organisations and institutions where people gather.

Workplaces

The workplace provides a favourable framework for health promotion. As Chu et al. (1997) observe, an infrastructure and organisation exist within workplaces for coordinating and developing programs that in turn are more likely to be successful and of low cost (and therefore more sustainable) than programs without infrastructure.

In general, health promotion programs in the workplace are distinct and separate from the responsibilities that employers have in the implementation of proper occupational health and safety measures. They include such activities as testing, health screening, ergonomics, education, provision of physical facilities such as fitness centres, ongoing health checks and occupational programs specific to particular industries.

Although the rationale for workplace health promotion would seem apparent, outcomes are not always so obvious. The provision of fitness facilities in many workplaces in Australia is often not successful, as they are often used by only a small number of dedicated staff (Giles-Corti & Donovan 2002, 2003). Unlike the USA, where corporations have a financial incentive for providing health services to staff, Australian corporations often have difficulty persuading staff that the workplace is more than a place to visit for a set time to complete their work requirements.

Workplace health promotion might also be condoned but not supported by a supervisor. Workers might feel coerced to participate by management. From a business perspective, both the direct and the indirect costs of the program must be considered and those with influence in a corporation convinced that improvements to the revenue base of the company are likely to result. Workplace health promotion programs might create disruptions in work scheduling and can create employee relations problems. For these and other reasons, results from evaluations of workplace health promotion interventions are often mixed (Heaney & Goetzel 1997).

Despite these difficulties, health promotion in the workplace—by addressing deficits in knowledge, choice and social support in relation to a range of healthy behaviour—does hold promise for improving employee health, and has the potential to reduce social inequalities in health. A stimulus to this would be government and workplace regulations requiring minimum health promotion inputs for staff as part of occupational health requirements, a situation that already exists in some areas, such as providing workplace smoking policies and smoking cessation programs.

Health promoting schools

School health promotion has grown significantly from a narrow concept focused on health instruction in the classroom to a much broader framework. Booth and Samdal (1997) characterise health promoting schools under six domains of activity, emphasising that, in practice, these domains should be as thoroughly integrated as possible:

- the formal curriculum
- school ethos (the social environment)
- the physical environment
- the policies and practices of the school
- school health services, and
- school–home–community interaction.

As might be anticipated, the adoption of a holistic health promoting school concept is not achievable overnight. However, where implementation of programs is strategic and structured, gains can be made. An example of this approach can be found in the Western Australian School Health Project (WASH Project), in which school-based health committees introduced practical health strategies while also developing longer-term health promotion action

Case study 7.5

ACTIVE-ATE: A program to promote healthy eating and activity in primary schools

The Active-Ate program is delivered largely via an active web site to Queensland primary schools (www.health.qld.gov.au/activeate), although some materials are delivered by mail. The program involves a wide range of activities summarised under the headings shown in the jigsaw. This is now one of a large number of programs targeting school-age children with healthy lifestyle interventions.

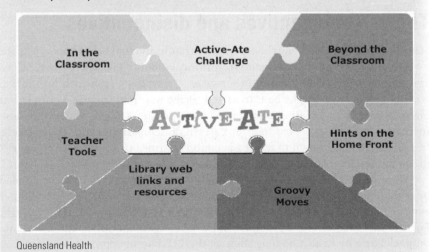

Queensland Health

plans for each school (Cameron & McBride 1995). Some of the achievements of the WASH Project included:

- changes in individual participants (e.g. a significant increase in teacher and parent knowledge and their self-reported use of health promotion strategies)
- school health promotion activities (e.g. a significant increase in school-wide health promotion events, such as healthy breakfasts), and
- school structural changes for health promotion (e.g. a significant increase in schools writing health policies, forming health committees, developing healthy canteens).

In another study, which looked at school policy effects on smoking in schoolchildren in Western Australia, Hamilton, O'Connell and Cross (2003) found that the actions taken to deal with students who violate smoking policy restrictions could be more important in reducing cigarette smoking than the presence of health or drug policies or health committees. Using education or counselling and discipline strategies rather than discipline only could help to reduce teenage smoking, showing the benefits of a combined approach.

As has been observed with workplace health promotion, the development of valid evaluation instruments—to measure program implementation and to assess the effects of health promoting school interventions—has lagged behind the development of conceptual and practical advances in this area (Booth & Samdal 1997). Nevertheless, the health promoting schools movement is a global one, consistent with WHO principles (WHO 1995), and provides an opportunity to influence positively the health of a target group of unquestionable importance in our society: our children.

The use of incentives and disincentives

Stimulus–response learning theory implies that individual behaviour is learned as a result of positive and negative reinforcements. The use of incentives and disincentives, economic or otherwise, is a strategy in health promotion with potential that might be unrealised. Price manipulation is a simple but obvious example. Taxation changes to food products—both reductions and increases—can be expected to alter patterns of consumption of those foods. In particular, it is known that in bad economic times the purchase of 'generic' food products increases, and the sale of known brands decreases.

Manipulation at the point of sale is an option that is relatively unused by nutritionists, even though commercial research shows that up to 50 per cent of food sale decisions are made at this point (Donovan & Henley 2004). Further incentives in food purchase include the introduction of endorsements on packaging by health bodies, such as the NHF food approval program (see case study 7.6).

Changes in demand for such substances as alcohol and tobacco can also be significantly affected by price increases resulting from sales and excise taxes. Australia is unique in its funding of health promotion programs in several states through a special levy on tobacco. This has allowed anti-smoking sponsorships of sport, which might have otherwise received tobacco sponsorship money (see case study 7.8).

Case study 7.6

A credible endorsement incentive—the National Heart Foundation's food approval program

In 1989 the National Heart Foundation of Australia (NHF) introduced its food approval program—'Pick the Tick'—to consumers and industry (Schrapnel 1993). The program provides NHF endorsement for foods that meet criteria for good health as laid down by an expert panel of the NHF, and for which industry pays an endorsement fee. The fee is invested in the program's administration and promotion and in related nutrition education initiatives. The NHF is also planning to establish a new Nutrition Research Fund to be funded by food approval program licence fees.

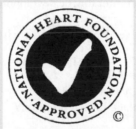

The food approval program is based on consumer research, which shows that shoppers are becoming increasingly conscious of the need for healthy eating but are still confused about appropriate food selections.

As a postscript, a similar food-labelling scheme, the Heart Guide program introduced by the American Heart Association (AHA) in the USA—which used a red heart symbol on selected foods—had to be withdrawn after pressure from disadvantaged food industry interests finally led to intervention by the Food and Drug Administration. The AHA is now seeking alternative ways to improve shoppers' food selection skills.

The idea of food labelling has merit, but it is difficult to operate and requires the cooperation and agreement of health, nutrition and industry groups. Although generally supporting the NHF food approval 'tick', public health authorities still hold some concerns about it. The main concern appears to be that, as the current program involves a 'fee-for-service', processed foods (including oils) feature more prominently than unprocessed foods (such as fresh fruit and vegetables). Ideally such a program should drive total food consumption patterns rather than favour certain categories of foods.

Schrapnel 1993

Major changes in taxation policy obviously require detailed negotiations. Introduction of tax changes is difficult for governments concerned about possible electoral backlash. At the local level, the health promotion practitioner can facilitate incentives, such as in local food outlets. Approaches can be made to cooperative supermarket managers with the incentive of increasing sales of healthy foods (e.g. fruits and vegetables, breakfast cereals, low-fat dairy products) through such initiatives as:

- in-store promotions
- having a nutritionist on the spot, and
- changing point-of-sale materials.

Manufacturers are also often keen to be involved in promotions that positively affect the sales of their products. Increased interest in health in recent times has created a market for the development of products specifically with a health orientation.

Economic incentives have also been used with individuals

- to encourage smokers at the workplace to quit smoking
- to reduce sickness absenteeism
- to help people lose weight, and
- to be involved in workplace health programs.

Sponsorship

'Sponsorship' is generally defined as payment for the right to associate the sponsor's company name, products or services with a 'sponsee' in return for various promotional benefits to the sponsor. The sponsee might be:

- an organisation—for example the NHF being sponsored by a drug company
- an event—for example a triathlon
- a series of events—for example a theatre season
- an individual—for example a prominent sports person, or
- a group of individuals—for example an AFL team.

Many high-profile commercial sponsorships are accompanied by extensive promotional activities, such as mass media advertising, product samplings, trade promotions and exclusive merchandising agreements (Phillips 1994).

SEAL: Supportive Environments for Active Living

SEAL is a government initiative providing a framework for state and local government personnel and non-government organisations to engage strategically in planning together with the community for the creation, enhancement and sustainability of environments that support active living.

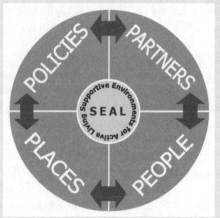

Queensland Health

- The SEAL Policies element provides the 'big picture' foundation for sustainable initiatives.
- The SEAL Partners element outlines a collaborative partnership approach to interventions.
- The SEAL People element outlines community engagement and participatory processes to improve vertical and horizontal social capital and build community spirit.
- The SEAL Places element provides the necessary guidelines for planning, designing and enhancing the physical environment to deliver safe and supportive active living opportunities.

The SEAL Strategic Framework for Action is available online at www.health.qld.gov.au/phs/Documents/sphun/13331.pdf

Sponsorship is considered to offer a number of benefits or opportunities to the sponsor:

- the ability to reach specific target audiences cost-effectively with little wastage on people outside the target group (e.g. young people at rock concerts; joggers at a fun run)

Case study 7.8

Sponsorship and the Health Promotion Foundations— the case of Healthway

The advent of tobacco tax-funded health promotion foundations is a relatively new phenomenon in public health theory and practice. In Australia, foundations now exist in two states; the first (VicHealth) having been established in 1987 in Victoria. Interest in the concept of health promotion foundations is now spreading to other parts of the globe and Carroll (1993, 2003) has now documented the Australian and overseas experiences for adoption in other countries.

Although no two of the Australian foundations are identical, the following description of the Western Australian Health Promotion Foundation (known as 'Healthway') illustrates the principal concepts. Healthway was established in 1991 under tobacco control legislation that outlawed the public promotion of tobacco products. Healthway is funded by a levy raised on the wholesale distribution of tobacco products. It uses approximately 60 per cent of its funds to sponsor sport, arts and racing groups (SARGs)—racing including horse, greyhound and motor-car racing. SARGs could range from one-off small craft exhibitions to a series of State Theatre plays, or from coaching clinics for junior soccer players to professional league teams such as AFL and National Basketball League teams.

When Healthway provides sponsorship funds (a 'grant') to a SARG, it simultaneously awards support funds to an independent health agency to promote a health message at the sport, arts or racing event. Health organisations (e.g. the NHF, Cancer Foundation, Diabetes Association) and their messages (e.g. 'Be Smoke Free', 'Be Active Every Day', 'Eat More Fruit and Veg.', 'Be Sun Wise', 'Drinksafe') are chosen primarily with respect to the nature of the particular event's audience or participants, and with respect to the state's health priority areas. For very small grants, and especially for country SARGs, rather than allocating funds to a health agency, Healthway provides the SARG with a sponsorship support kit containing posters, pamphlets and ideas for activities related to a specific health message.

Healthway also attempts to create healthy environments at the event by negotiating the introduction of smoke-free areas, availability of low-alcohol and non-alcohol alternatives, safe alcohol serving practices, provision of healthy food choices and sun protection measures (such as shaded spectator areas and protective clothing). These initiatives are the equivalent of merchandising and stocking agreements in commercial sponsorship. Healthway also provides grants for research projects (approximately 10 per cent of funds) and for community interventions (approximately 30 per cent). In 1994–5 Healthway distributed approximately $12 million.

Carroll 2003

- the opportunity for potential trial of the sponsor's product where the sponsorship includes exclusive stocking agreements (e.g. a soft drink or snack-food marketer)
- hospitality for clients, employees and other stakeholders
- the generation of community goodwill by sponsoring not-for-profit organisations popular with the community, and
- enhanced communication effects, such as increased company profile, increased brand awareness and brand image formation or reinforcement associated with positive attributes of the sponsored event or individual (Sweeny 1992).

The sponsee also benefits in a number of ways, including the raising of the organisation's profile in the community—an important benefit for non-profit organisations' fundraising efforts—and the attraction of members or volunteers (Donovan et al. 1993). For sponsored health organisations, the major benefits are the increased ability to promote their health messages to a larger number of people and to reach target audiences who might not otherwise be reached (Corti et al. 1997).

In most countries, total sponsorship expenditure is still minuscule relative to other marketing expenditure, but this figure is increasing and is expected to grow at an increasing rate. Growth is being fuelled by the increased costs of media and other promotions, and by the apparent cost-effectiveness of sponsorship—at least in terms of delivering media exposure of the sponsor's brand name or logo for a minimal outlay.

The entry of large companies into sponsorship programs has also been stimulated by non-profit organisations actively promoting themselves as vehicles for sponsorship (e.g. the Australian Institute of Sport and Kellogg's 'Sustain', and the NHF's 'tick' labelling).

Sponsorship, particularly of sport, received major impetus in Australia as a result of the tobacco companies seeking ways to continue to promote their brands following bans on television advertising and, later, on other forms of promotion (Chapman & Lupton 1994). Given the tobacco companies' apparent success in maintaining brand awareness and image via sponsorship, other companies—led by the major brewery and soft drink marketers— have increasingly included sponsorship in their promotional mix.

During this same period, health promotion professionals adopted many of the concepts and tools of commercial marketing, and now are enthusiastically embracing sponsorship, both as sponsors (mainly government agencies) and by actively promoting themselves to business as sponsees (non-government agencies).

The growth in health sponsorship has been facilitated in Australia primarily by the health promotion foundations. The growth in health sponsorship has been facilitated further by the deliberate policy in some states of guaranteeing the replacement of tobacco sponsorship funds with health promotion foundation funds following the legislative phasing out of tobacco sponsorship.

Does sponsorship work?

In January 1992 the University of Western Australia was commissioned by Healthway to undertake the Health Promotion Development and Evaluation Program (HPDEP) over a period of three years. HPDEP, a joint undertaking of the Graduate School of Management and the Department of Public Health, is now known as the Health Promotion Evaluation Unit (HPEU). Through HPDEP/HPEU, Healthway has carried out extensive evaluation of its sponsorship activities (Corti et al. 1997; Donovan et al. 1997; Holman et al. 1996). Generally, these evaluations show that sponsorship can be effective in increasing awareness of health messages and in creating intentions to adopt healthy behaviour.

A healthy environment—ecological considerations

The union of health promotion and concern for the natural environment is an idea whose time has come. Environmental changes have traditionally been one of the cornerstones of public health: the provision of potable water, garbage disposal and sanitation. In the past, these modifications have been made to a hostile natural environment that Western tradition has felt obliged to tame. Ironically, when this appears to have been achieved, the environment has fought back in an unexpected and potentially more dangerous way.

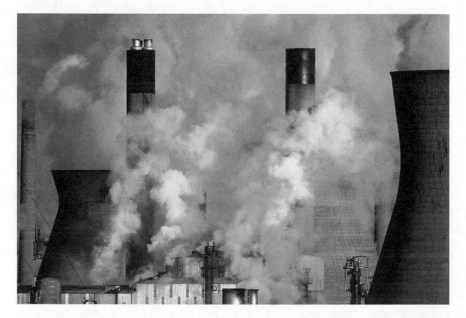

Photo Library

Dubos (1988) expressed his concern for the current predicament of the human race in the following way:

> In short, the two worlds of man [sic]—the biosphere of his inheritance, the technosphere of his creation—are out of balance, indeed potentially in deep conflict. And man is in the middle. This is the hinge of history at which we stand, the door of the future opening on to a crisis more sudden, more global, more inescapable, and more bewildering than any ever encountered by the human species and one which will take decisive shape within the life span of children who are already born.

Environmental degradation, pollution, the greenhouse effect, disappearance of the ozone layer and the disruption of the world's ecosystem have all become apparent as a result of attempts to improve living standards. They pose future challenges not only to scientists and politicians but also to health workers and educationists. After all, it is likely to be changes in human behaviour—in population growth, resource use and economic activity—that will stop environmental degradation over the long term. To this end, the health promotion practitioner of the future is likely to work with environmentalists, engineers and ecologists.

Without close consideration, it might be expected that the contributions of health science and technological development to humanity would all be positive. In his epic novel *Brave New World*, Aldous Huxley questioned this as being what he called 'the myth of progress'. In essence, Huxley saw all medical and scientific advances as a danger to the human race because each of them promotes the survival and propagation of the biologically and genetically unfit. These advances then negate the forces of natural selection and might ultimately be responsible for the fall of humanity.

As early as 1964, Boulding related the development of negative returns in health to the exponential growth of human populations: '... if the only thing which can check the growth of population is starvation and misery, then the population will grow until it is sufficiently miserable and starving to check its own growth' (Boulding 1964).

Taking this argument further, the Club of Rome, in its report *The Limits to Growth* (1974), reported on a computer simulation of energy usage and exponential growth of world population. It concluded that major catastrophe would occur to the environment early in the twenty-first century if major changes in the direction of resource use were not made immediately. The response to this prediction was typically one of cynicism with futurists reverting to history to demonstrate that dire predictions in the past (e.g. about the proliferation of horse manure that would occur with growth in population) were always solved by technical ingenuity. Few could see that the Club of Rome's predictions might be reflected in alterations in the ozone and carbon-dioxide levels in the environment, or global warming in the time period predicted; all of which have the potential for major changes in the world's environment and human health.

Population growth is an obvious area of concern to all involved in human health and services. Whereas it took from the beginning of the human race's time on Earth to 1850 for the world population to reach a billion, it required only another hundred years for that number to double. On present trends, the number will double again in the first two decades of the twenty-first century. And, although population growth has slowed in the developed world, there is no indication of slower growth in those parts of the world where demand for the earth's resources has yet to increase. Population control and family planning will obviously become major roles for the preventive health worker of the future. This poses a range of religious, philosophical and democratic challenges, which will need to be addressed.

However, population growth alone might be merely a symptom of a more deep-seated and insidious cause. The drive for economic growth at an exponential rate—which is required in current Western economies—means either that more resources must be consumed per person, more people must exist to consume more resources or new resources must be discovered or produced more efficiently. The combination of resource depletion and population growth creates an environmental time bomb that might eventually require a major paradigm shift in the way in which we live. As pointed out by Morrison (2003) in *Plague Species*, a book about runaway growth,

> We have dallied too long at the banquet of natural resources, only to discover that the only way out is past the cashier. Even among those who are aware of the scale of our environmental debt, the general consensus seems to be that with the aid of a little fast technological tap dancing most of us may make our escape without paying the full price. Not only would this involve a drastic and immediate reduction in the daily rate at which we gobble up the world's energy resources and dump our wastes, but we would have to sacrifice two of western civilization's most sacred cows—Growth and Progress—to do it.

Without a consideration of all this in health promotion, the health promotion practitioner could be 'cooking dinner while the house is burning' (Dunnette 1989).

A new challenge for health promotion in the twenty-first century will be dealing with the consequences of the ecological disruptions that are already occurring throughout the world. This has been summed up eloquently by Australian epidemiologist Dr Tony McMichael in the following way:

> ... a new and unfamiliar public health hazard is emerging. The fact that the hazard is neither immediate nor tangible is part of the problem. This is a qualitatively different category of public health problem from those previously encountered. Much of it is global in scope; it does not depend on directly acting environmental exposures; it transcends generations; and some aspects may be irreversible. It includes global warming and its many ecological consequences, increased exposure to biologically damaging ultra-violet radiation, loss of arable land, destruction of parts of our food chain, loss of biodiversity, and urban

crowding and social disintegration. While there is much that is uncertain and controversial, there is little doubt that recent trends and their implications for human health are troubling. (McMichael 1992)

McMichael's warning is not a doomsday prophecy. He observes that an ecological transition to a sustainable society could be achieved if we breathe life into the much-parroted phrase 'our common future': 'The stabilisation of resource use, and of human numbers, will require radical reforms of our core values, economic priorities and structures—and of social decision-making processes. It will require governments, private enterprise, non-government organisations, communities and economists—we're all in this together.' (McMichael & Hales 1997)

Furthermore, as we undertake some of the above reforms we should not underestimate the role of public health measures in combating at least some of the problems that we face. For example some authorities have expressed concern that all the attention to global warming as a public health problem could distract the public from other, more urgent, health priorities.

Implications for the health promotion practitioner

How can the health promotion practitioner influence such broad issues as the natural environment?

In the first place, health promotion skills can assist with awareness of the problem as it relates to health. Media acceptance of environmental problems has now allowed a forum for this discussion to take place. The relationship of environmental issues to health is apparent not only in obvious ways (e.g. exposure to sunlight and potential increases in skin cancer) but also in less obvious ways (e.g. pollution). Awareness needs to be translated into knowledge, which can be converted into action. This requires action at all levels of intervention—using the media, community organisation and community development—in an approach that incorporates global—not just local—thinking. Action might not simply involve changing individual behaviour but might involve mobilising against major forces of opposition in the environment, such as non-renewable resource industries.

Methods for modifying the health environment

Because the role of the health promotion practitioner in environmental interventions has no well-defined professional precedents, there are no clear rules of operation. However, some principles include the following:

- investigation and communication concerning local environmental issues and problems that influence health
- political lobbying at the local as well as national and State levels
- letter writing, including deputation-style letters for constituents' signatures
- community organisation at several levels of involvement

- community development, particularly among affected groups and individuals
- awareness raising, by use of the media, public forums, lectures, organised debates, article writing, publicity and festivals
- demonstration–participation programs, for example clean-ups, smoke-outs, live-ins, and
- cooperation with local retailers, wholesalers and manufacturers for mutually advantageous gains, including sponsorships.

Summary of environmental adaptations

Manipulations of the health environment often represent the greatest challenge to the health practitioner, but can also be the most cost-effective and time-effective processes for influencing health behaviour. Even though the focus is macro-level change, the issues at stake pose considerably greater potential risk to life and health for the community than do individual risk factors.

Because the basis of much ill-health in modern times lies in structural and sociopolitical causes, it is important for the health promotion practitioner to attempt to modify these causes at the local or national level. The Greenpeace motto 'Think globally, act locally' is an apt principle for operation at this level. Doing so could involve the use of any or all of the strategies outlined above. But it could also involve a creative approach to more direct action.

Career opportunities in health promotion

Environmental interventions have always been a part of effective public health, albeit from a different perspective than is required today. Health promotion practitioners have potential opportunities in an entrepreneurial capacity, such as in designing, promoting and selling 'active technology' like fitness equipment, active games and so on. Politics and political lobbying offer other opportunities, as does employment as environmental health or sport and recreation officers with local councils. Teaching is also expanding in the area of personal development and physical education in schools, and there is a requirement for nutrition consultants and advisers for establishing and running school tuckshops. Health promotion personnel working in community development or family planning also stimulate much environmental change, particularly in developing countries. Specialists in injury prevention and public health workers are often also required to have a background in health promotion.

References

Bevins, J., 1988, 'Reducing communication abuse', paper presented to the 4th Drug Education Conference, Perth, WA

Bierer, M. F., & Rigotti, N. A., 1992, 'Public policy for the control of tobacco-related disease', *Clin Med North Am* 76:515–39.

Booth, M. L., & Samdal, O., 1997, 'Health-promoting schools in Australia: models and measurement', *Aust NZ J Pub Health* 21(4):365–70.

Boulding, K., 1964, *The Meaning of the Twentieth Century*, Harper & Row, New York.

Brownell, K. D., 2004, *Food Fight*, Contemporary Books, New York.

Cameron, L., & McBride, N., 1995, 'Creating health promoting schools: lessons from the Western Australian School Health Project', *Health Prom J Aust* 5(1):4–10.

Campkin, H., 1990, 'The cost of traffic accidents', paper presented to the Federal Office of Road Safety Conference on Road Safety, Canberra.

Carroll, A., 1993, 'The Western Australian Health Promotion Foundation—Healthway', *Health Prom J Aust* 3:42–3.

—— 2003, *Taxing Sin for Health: A Report Commissioned by the Western Pacific Regional Office of the World Health Organization*, WHO, Geneva.

Chapman, S., 2004, 'Public health advocacy', in Moodie, R., & Hulme, A. (eds), *Hands-on Health Promotion*, IP Communications, Melbourne,Vic.

Chapman, S., Borland, R., Hill, D., Owen, N., & Woodward, S., 1990, 'Why the tobacco industry fears the passive smoking issue', *Int J Health Serv* 20(3):417–27.

Chapman, S., & Lupton, D., 1994, *The Fight for Public Health: Principles and Practices of Media Advocacy*, BMJ Books, London.

Chu, C., Driscoll, T., & Dwyer, S., 1997, 'The health-promoting workplace: an integrative perspective', *Aust NZ J Pub Health* 21(4):377–85.

Club of Rome, 1974, *The Limits to Growth*, Universe Books, New York.

Corti, B., Holman, C. D. J., Donovan, R. J., Frizzell, S. K., & Carroll, A. M., 1997, 'Using sponsorship to promote health messages to children', *Health Educ & Behav* 24(3):276–86.

Donovan, R. J., Corti, B., Holman, C. D. J., West, D., & Pitter, D., 1993, 'Evaluating sponsorship effectiveness', *Health Prom J Aust* (3):63–7.

Donovan, R. J., & Henley, N., 2003, *Social Marketing: Principles and Practice*, IP Communications, Melbourne.

Donovan, R. J., Holman, C. D. J., Corti, B., & Jalleh, G., 1997, 'Evaluating sponsorship effectiveness: an epidemiological approach to analysing survey data', *Australasian J Market Res* 6:9–23.

Dubos, R., 1988, *Only One Earth*, Doubleday, London.

Dunnette, D. A., 1989, 'Cooking dinner while the house is burning: an environmental scientist's view of health education needs for the 1990s', *Health Ed* 20(7):4–7.

Eckstrand, J., 1989, 'Effectiveness of a sports injury prevention program', paper presented to the First World Conference on Injury Prevention, Stockholm, Sweden.

Elkington, J. M., Carey, V., & Fowler, D., 1992, 'Public perceptions of the New South Wales pool fencing legislation', *Health Prom J Aust* 2(1):34–7.

Egger, G., & Swinburn, B., 1997, 'An ecological approach to the obesity pandemic', *Brit Med J* 315:477–80.

Egger, G., Swinburn, B., & Rossner, S., 2002, 'Dusting off the epidemiological triad: could it work with obesity?', *Obes Rev* 3:289–301.

Giles-Corti, B., & Donovan, R., 2002, 'The relative influence of individual, social and physical environmental determinants of physical activity', *Social Science and Medicine* 54:1793–812.

—— 2003, 'Increasing walking: the relative influence of individual, social environment and physical environmental factors', *Am J Pub Health* 93(9):1583–9.

Haddon, W., 1980, 'Advances in the epidemiology of injuries as a basis for public policy', *Pub Health Rep* 95(5):411–20.

Hamilton, G., O'Connell, M., & Cross, D., 2003, 'Adolescent smoking cessation: development of a school nurse intervention', *J Sch Nurs* 20(3):169–74.

Harris, E., & Wills, J., 1997, 'Developing healthy communities at local government level: lessons from the past decade', *Aust NZ J Pub Health* 21(4):403–12.

Heaney, C. A., & Goetzel, R. Z., 1997, 'A review of health-related outcomes of multi-component worksite health promotion programs', *Amer J Health Prom* 11(4):290–307.

Holman, C. D. J., Donovan, R. J., Corti, B., Jalleh, G., Frizzell, S. K., & Carroll, A. M., 1996, 'Evaluating projects funded by the Western Australian Health Promotion Foundation: first results', *Health Prom Int* 11(2):75–88.

Kickbush, I., 1997, 'Health promoting environments: the next steps', *Aust NZ J Pub Health* 21(4):431–4.

McCarthy, W. H., & Shaw, A. M., 1989, 'Skin cancer in Australia', *Medical Journal of Australia* 150:469.

McMichael, A., 1992, 'Ecological disruption and human health: the next great challenge to public health', *Aust J Pub Health* 16(1):3–5.

McMichael, A., & Hales, S., 1997, 'Global health promotion: looking back to the future', *Aust NZ J Pub Health* 21(4):425–8.

Mock, C., Quansah, R., Krishnan, R., Arreola-Risa, C., & Rivara, F., 2004, 'Strengthening the prevention and care of injuries worldwide', *Lancet* 363:2172–9.

Morley-John, J., Swinburn, B., Metcalf, P., Raza, F., & Wright, H., 2002, 'Fat content of chips, quality of frying fat and deep-frying practices in New Zealand fast food outlets', *Aust NZ J Public Health* 26:101–7.

Morrison, R., 2003, *Plague Species: Is It In Our Genes?*, Reed New Holland, Sydney.

Nutbeam, D., 1997, 'Creating health-promoting environments: overcoming barriers to action', *Aust NZ J Pub Health* 21(4):355–9.

Oliver, T., & Lawson, J., 1979, 'Glass laceration injuries and prevention', *M J Aust* 1:90.

Phillips, M., 1994, 'Does sponsorship pay?', *Marketing* 48:12–17.

Pierce, J. P., Evans, N., Farkas, A., Cavin, S. W., & Beery, C., 1994, *Tobacco Use in California: An Evaluation of the Tobacco Control Program 1989–93*, University of California, San Diego.

Sallis, J. F., & Owen, N., 1996, 'Ecological models', in Glanz, K., Lewis, F. M., & Rimer, B. K. (eds), *Health Behaviour and Health Education: Theory, Research and Practice*, Jossey-Bass, San Francisco, pp. 403–24.

Schelp, L., 1987, 'Community intervention and changes in accident pattern in a rural Swedish municipality', *Health Prom* 2(2):109–25.

Schrapnel, W. S., 1993, 'The National Heart Foundation "Pick the Tick" Program: nutrition labelling and supermarket promotions to encourage healthy food choices', *Health Prom J Aust* 3(2):36–8.

Sleet, D., 1990, 'Injury prevention', seminar presentation to the Western Australian Professional Health Education Association (WAPHEA), Perth.

Steckler, A., Allegrante, J. P., Altman, D., Brown, R., Burdine, J. N., Goodman, R. M., & Jorgensen, C. J., 1995, 'Health education intervention strategies: recommendations for future research', *Health Ed Quart* 22(3):307–28.

Sweeney, B., 1992, *Australians and Sport*, Brian Sweeney & Associates, Melbourne, Vic.

Swinburn, B., 2002, 'Influencing environments to reduce obesity prevalence', plenary paper presented to the 9th International Congress on Obesity, Sao Paulo, Brazil.

Swinburn, B., Egger, G., & Raza, F., 1999, 'Dissecting obesogenic environments: part of a public health approach to reducing obesity', *Prev Med* 29:563–70.

Thompson, D., & Rivara, F., 2003, 'Pool fencing for preventing drowning in children', in *The Cochrane Library*, Issue 1, Update Software, Oxford.

US Department of Health and Human Services, 1994, *Preventing Tobacco Use Among Young People: A Report of the Surgeon General*, US Government Printing Office, Washington, DC.

Vogels, N., Plaqui, G., Egger, G., & Westerterp, K., 2004, 'Secular trends in physical activity: implications for health inventions', *Int J Sports Med* Nov 2004.

WHO (World Health Organization), 1986, *Ottawa Charter for Health Promotion*, International Conference on Health Promotion, Ottawa.

—— 1995, *WHO Expert Committee on Comprehensive School Health Education and Promotion*, WHO, Geneva.

Chapter 8
Factors influencing strategy selection

Summary of main points

- The selection of the right strategy in health promotion can depend on a range of factors, including the intended recipients, temporal factors, program factors and the level of community acceptance and participation.
- Strategy selection can also be influenced by the rate at which ideas are diffused among an intended audience.
- Different strategies might be needed to reach an audience with low economic means and who are at high risk.
- Although a strategy might be applicable in particular circumstances, combinations of strategies are usually required.
- Health promotion strategies that ignore the deeper social causes of ill-health are unlikely to be successful over the long term.
- Obtaining ongoing funding for health promotion will be dependent on evaluated successful outcomes.

An understanding of all the processes discussed to this point should lead to the following conclusions:

- that the professional health promotion practitioner, by necessity, needs to be a specialist in generalisation
- that knowledge is required in both the content of health issues and the processes by which change can be instigated to attain health gains
- that the three most common words in discussing the relevance of health promotion strategies are 'it all depends'
- that the role of the health promotion practitioner is often that of a translator (translating information from the scientific community to the general public), a moderator, a facilitator and/or a catalyst for action
- that the understanding of one's limitations and development of one's skills in the range of strategies available is of prime professional concern to the health promotion practitioner

- that strategies for coping with individual risk are important, but should not be used to the neglect of strategies dealing with lowering average risk in whole communities and addressing risk conditions, as well as risk factors that predispose to ill-health, and
- that all strategies are valid and potentially useful, and that combinations of strategies and methods are likely to yield the best results.

The approach taken here has been strategies- and methods-based rather than settings-based. The application of strategies and methods to settings is one that requires the knowledge and experience of the practitioner and an appreciation of the needs of the target group. For example:

- *school-based programs*: can include the lecture–discussion format and any or all of the different group methods or broader health-promoting schools approaches
- *workplace programs*: could call for group techniques, plus risk factor analysis and changes to the workplace environment (such as workstations and healthy canteens)
- *institution-based programs* (e.g. hospitals): could involve aspects of group and individual focus as well as community organisation processes
- *local action programs*: might be centred on community development but also involve individual and group methods where appropriate
- *large-scale community programs*: could use the media and social marketing as an umbrella, but include group and individual processes, capacity building and partnership arrangements as part of community organisation.

Case study 8.1

Detailing success in health promotion

Successes

An analysis of achievements in health promotion (NH&MRC 1996) shows that at least half of the more than 30 per cent decline in all cause mortality in Australia from the 1960s has been owing to prevention. Most notable are:

- the decrease in male smoking from 75 per cent in 1945 to 22 per cent in 2002, resulting in a 20 per cent drop in lung cancer and decreases in heart disease
- a 33 per cent drop in deaths from traffic crashes from the peak in 1970 to 1994
- a 70 per cent decrease in cyclists killed or with a head injury
- a 30 per cent reduction in mortality owing to cancer of the cervix
- a 63 per cent decease in cardiovascular disease since the peak in 1968

- a decrease in incidence and deaths from AIDS/HIV since its beginnings in 1980.

Lessons

The lessons learned from this have been that good health promotion requires:

1. use of multiple and comprehensive strategies
2. intersectoral collaboration
3. active leadership of the health sector
4. sound epidemiological data informing of the nature and extent of the problem
5. quality research on the effectiveness of interventions, and monitoring and surveillance
6. political commitment and clear goals
7. workforce development and training
8. high-level and widespread advocacy
9. sustainability of approaches.

Barriers

Barriers needing to be overcome include:

1. lack of leadership on any particular health issue
2. lack of coordination of different levels of government
3. uncontrolled advertising and promotion of competitive, unhealthy, products and services
4. lack of quality information and detailed planning to guide action
5. public apathy or antagonism to change.

Selecting strategies

The selection of a health promotion strategy can vary depending on:

- the intended recipients
- temporal factors (i.e. whether a society is historically ready for such change)
- program factors in the delivery of the programs, and
- the level of community acceptance and participation.

In advanced industrialised cultures, many changes occur in social and health behaviour before, and independent of, planned health promotion initiatives. The fitness boom of the 1970s, for example, and the tremendous increases in interest in nutrition and the environment in the 1980s and 1990s could not realistically be ascribed to any planned health input. By their very nature of detailed planning and organisation, health promotion activities normally climb onto a wave of public reaction rather than start that wave. What determines the initial wave is the subject of much scientific speculation, but geopolitical, economic and demographic forces are as important as any developments in health science.[1]

Case study 8.2

Five large-scale prevention studies that have worked

Although not everything works in health promotion, it is useful to take the lessons from those projects where it does. Some prominent examples include the following:

1. A four-year project in California from 1989 to 1992 used mass media and programs based in the community, schools and worksites to reduce smoking. There were 33 000 fewer deaths from heart disease in that time than would have been expected on the basis of previous trends (Fichtenberg & Glantz 2000).
2. In Finland, half of a group of 522 middle-aged, overweight men at risk of developing diabetes received individualised counselling about reducing weight, improving diet and increasing physical activity over six years (Uusitupa et al. 2003). At the end of the trial 58 per cent fewer of the (lifestyle) intervention group had developed diabetes than the control group (no lifestyle intervention). Importantly, these effects have been maintained over three years (Lindstrom et al. 2003).
3. In the USA a larger study of 3225 men and women at risk of developing diabetes undertook a lifestyle change program (150 minutes physical activity per week plus weight reduction) over four years, compared with a group on a diabetes drug (Metformin) and a control group. Fifty-eight per cent fewer in the lifestyle group compared to controls progressed to diabetes compared to 33 per cent in the drug group (Knowler et al. 2002).
4. In the Torres Strait (Australia) a diabetes outreach service improved care outcomes for diabetics, but an effective community-based register, managed by local health workers, was critical to its success. It reduced diabetes-related hospitalisations by 40 per cent in one year (McDermott et al. 2001).
5. In a sample of schools in the south-west of England an educational program aimed at reducing the consumption of carbonated soft drinks resulted in a decrease in soft drink intake as well as a significant reduction in weight gain over a year in test schools compared with controls (James et al. 2004).

In an early approach to dealing with the take-up of a health promotion program, Green and McAlister (1984) made indications about strategy selection based on the diffusion process. The basis of this approach is that the adoption of ideas in a community diffuses among individuals in that community at varying rates. Early in the introduction of a new idea, 'innovators' and 'early adopters', who are typically more affluent and keyed into national information networks, pick it up. 'Early' and 'late' majorities are next, and these people attend less to national media and more to local media, although they respond less to the media in general. The last group to adopt a new idea are called 'late adopters', and they are considered to be the hardest to reach.

This suggests different strategies at different phases of the adoption process, as shown in figure 8.1.

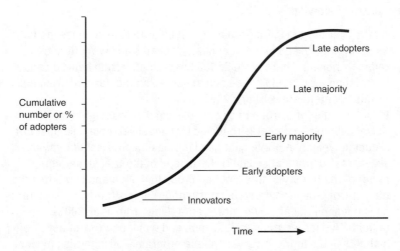

Figure 8.1: Diffusion of innovation process

The use of the mass media might be sufficient for adoption of ideas among innovators and early adopters; that is, early community leaders who are the social models for the majority. And although some analysts have indicated that the media alone are not sufficient to influence significant behaviour change (Redman, Spencer & Sanson-Fisher 1990), the effect of this group in determining and diffusing fashions and trends has been ignored or not adequately measured. Program factors have also not been included in evaluations of media, leading to questions and suggestions about their possible role.

Mass media, together with community organisation and capacity building processes, might be necessary to encourage change in the early and late majority. Because of its size, this should be the primary target group for most health promotion programs aimed at lowering average risk in populations. Organisational and institutional channels—such as those used in the Pawtucket Heart Health Study (Lasater, Carleton & LeFebvre 1988) and the North Karelia Project (Puska, Toumilehto & Salonen 1981)—are essential to the health promotion and social modelling strategies required to support changes in the behaviour of this group.

Community involvement and participation programs are necessary to reach late adopters, who are generally, but not always, of low economic means and high health risk. In developing countries, such strategies as community development form the core of health promotion activities with the media playing only a minor role.

Adoption of change

A second dimension is that of time between exposure and adoption. In line with diffusion theory, the stages of adoption from awareness to interest to trial to adoption occur at different rates of the diffusion process. There is a greater time-lag between phases at the late-adopter stage than at the early-adopter and innovator level.

Figure 8.2 shows the functions of the various interventions at different stages of the process. The media alone serve to influence behavioural outcomes among innovators, whereas it might be expected to create only awareness and interest in the early and late majority, and only interest among late adopters. Community organisation and on-the-ground programs begin to take effect at the trial-and-adoption phase in the early and late majority and at the awareness-and-interest phase in late adopters. Capacity building can occur at all levels. The use of the media with disadvantaged groups, in this case the late adopters, is often discredited, despite the fact that there have been few well-conducted studies.

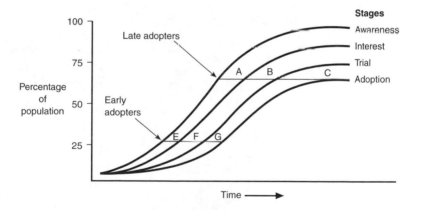

Figure 8.2: Time lapse between awareness, interest, trial and adoption

There is often an assumption that using the media is a 'top-down' strategy with middle-class messages being of little relevance to lower socioeconomic groups. This need not be the case, particularly if these groups have some control of the medium. The example of the locally based media associations controlled and run by Aborigines—such as the Central Australian Aboriginal Media Association (CAAMA)—demonstrates not only that the medium of television can be a useful channel for accessing hard-to-reach groups but also that the process of involvement can be one of empowerment for the groups concerned (Spark & Mills 1988).

It is important to remember that, although a specific strategy and/or method might be applicable in a particular circumstance, it might be necessary to combine strategies according to:

- the characteristics of the target group and their needs
- the type of intervention required
- the timeframe of the project
- the goals of the organisation sponsoring the project, and
- resources available, both financial and human.

Case study 8.3

A creative approach to nutrition education

The documentary film *Super Size Me* released in 2004 has had a seminal effect in changing attitudes to fast foods around the world, which shows the value of a creative approach to health promotion. Within months, several fast-food organisations had agreed to eliminate 'supersizing'—one of the main reasons for increases in food intake.

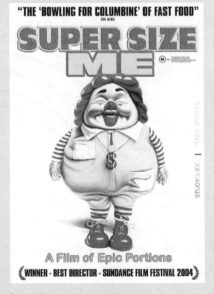

Dendy Films

To capitalise on the popularity of the documentary, a study guide became available via the Internet for use in schools.

What works for one health issue in one place for one period of time might not do so under other circumstances—'it all depends'. The skill in health promotion is in analysing and diagnosing—as well as in implementing—the appropriate strategies and methods of intervention (see chapter 9). For this reason, to be most effective, the health promotion practitioner should also be familiar with techniques of health promotion planning and program evaluation (see Hawe, Degeling & Hall 1990).

Issues for the future—economics and prevention

The days of a golden goose laying golden eggs in health promotion are long gone—if indeed they ever existed. Sponsoring bodies will not take it on trust that 'everyone will feel good' and that 'this intervention will reduce health costs in the future'. Sponsors now want to see hard data, or at least evidence that programs have been effective in relation to the investment made. Perhaps more than any other professional group, health promotion practitioners can feel vulnerable in the face of calls—frequently from other health professionals—to demonstrate the effectiveness of their programs. In a health system that is increasingly focused on evidence-based methods, health promotion practitioners need, at the very least, to be able to cite some of the evidence that does exist from individually focused interventions. They also need to develop instruments to evaluate the effectiveness of more complex interventions directed at settings or populations, such as community development interventions. For example, as Hawe et al. (1997) note:

> We have evidence from randomised controlled trials to show that health promotion interventions have brought about reductions in hypertension (Levine et al. 1979), and hospital readmission rates (Maiman et al. 1979), and increases in the proportion of people who quit smoking (Kotte et al. 1988), and who present for vaccination (Larson et al. 1982).

This issue has implications for the type of strategies selected and how strategy mixes are configured. The traditional focus of health promotion campaigns on individual risk should, by now, be just one part of total health promotion strategy. It is clear, according to Syme (1997), that multiple diseases appear to be linked to homogeneous groups of people.

Hence, interventions along the traditional lines of area specialisation might overlook co-existing health problems that have socioenvironmental roots. For example, in studies with bus drivers, Syme (1997) noted that this group suffered from high rates of a number of ailments, which might have been simply independent reactions to similar environmental factors: noise, stress, social environment, the 'tyranny of the schedule'. Strategies that focus on the total work environment rather than on individual disease causes could be more productive and more cost-effective. Therefore, to address the dilemma of the appropriate strategy selection for health promotion, useful advice for the health promotion practitioner is offered by Hawe and Sheil (1995), who advocate thinking about health promotion programs in the same way as one would conduct a prudent investment portfolio. This would range from blue-chip program investments (evaluated health promotion interventions where the likely impact is known)—such as cardiac patient education—through to higher-risk programs (i.e. higher uncertainty programs) but potentially high-gain investments—such as community capacity building and intersectoral health action.

Assessing needs

A needs assessment in a community is an obvious place to start when determining strategy selection. Needs can be assessed at a simple level by observation and situational analysis (see chapter 9) or more formally through quantitative surveys and epidemiological data collection. There is no hard and fast rule as to how this could be done, and different authors provide a variety of different approaches (Green & Kreuter 1999).

Case study 8.4

Creative outlets and the 'teachable moment'

Ignoring for a moment the ethics involved, drug manufacturers have been quick to capitalise on the 'teachable moment' to promote a new feminine product for comfortable sexual intercourse. This was done to counter the effects of adverse publicity about hormone replacement therapy (HRT) causing breast cancer. One drug company attempted to step into the breach for women concerned about not losing one of HRT's key selling points: more comfortable intercourse after menopause. Having realised that more menopausal women confide in their hairdressers than their doctors on these matters, the company used hairdressers to promote a new product, called Vagifem, for dealing with vaginal dryness. In a classic piece of 'disease-mongering', a web site about painful intercourse was used. Its address www.whylovehurts.com was emblazoned in reverse on hairdressers' capes, so their customers could see it while they sat in front of the mirror. Hairdressers also received scripted messages to use, along with fact sheets to hand out to customers. Sales of Vagifem spiked, and the ad agency concerned won the national award in the 'best one-off media campaign' for Australia.

Medical authorities were seeking to ban the promotion of drugs through these means.

Bastion 2002

One technique developed by the current authors is a 'component circuit' approach (Egger, Spark & Donovan 1990). This involves both qualitative and quantitative research (e.g. focus groups, semi-structured interviews, surveys and so on) in an iterative process, whereby results from one process feed forward to the next and then feed back after modification for verification. The process is shown graphically in case study 8.5.

Case study 8.5

Using a component circuit approach for needs assessment

A 'component circuit' approach (Egger, Spark & Donovan 1990), using quantitative (e.g. statistical and epidemiological data) and qualitative techniques (e.g. focus groups, interviews with experts, associations and so on) offers some structure to the process of needs assessment. This has been used, among other things, to estimate the costs of sports injuries in Australia (Egger 1991) and develop National Physical Activity Guidelines (Egger et al. 2001). The process and components of a typical circuit are shown in figure 8.3.

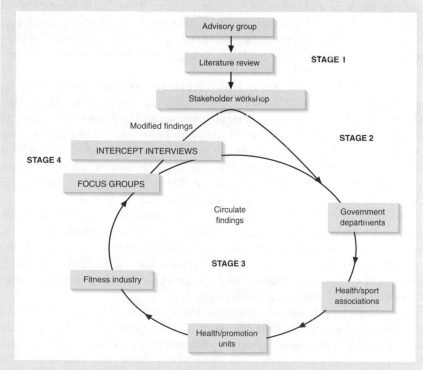

Figure 8.3: Components of a circuit for needs analysis

Counting the cost

The notion of cost-effectiveness is an important one that also needs to be addressed in the selection of strategies. Although it is often assumed that 'prevention is better than cure', this does not necessarily mean that it will be less costly in the long run. For example Russell (1986) claimed that successful health promotion in the early years could mean an increased number of aged people in the population who add to health costs in the later years. The philosophical dilemma here is one that can be resolved only when cost-effectiveness is compared with treatment costs in terms of outcome; that is, quality of life and potential years of life saved (Rogerson 1995). Cost/benefit is particularly important in introducing programs into industry. Unlike the USA, where health insurance is covered by employers, and where an incentive therefore exists to keep employee sickness costs to a minimum, there is little obvious incentive in Australian organisations.

Studies carried out in the USA show that sickness absenteeism can be reduced through the introduction of health promotion, and this can be translated into an economic bottom line for company managers. For example smokers have been reported to experience a 45 per cent greater rate of absenteeism than non-smokers and, according to Rentmeester (1984), cost a company an estimated average $650 per year ($1500 in 2004 prices) per smoking employee. The cost–benefit ratio for smoking cessation programs at the worksite has been estimated at 2:1; that is, for every dollar an employer invests in these programs, a two-dollar saving can be predicted.

Drug abuse is another area in which employers are now appreciating the economics of prevention. Based on US figures, alcoholism in Australian industry could be expected to cost employers around $2 billion per annum, and employer-based programs have been shown to be successful in reducing this cost. There is little data to quantify the increased productivity resulting from increased fitness and wellness of staff but, fortunately, large organisations such as Coles-Myer, Shell, Hewlett-Packard and IBM in Australia have not needed it to develop well-run programs in employee health.

Economics are also likely to become of increasing concern as the population ages. Health costs tend to increase for older people, who use medical services approximately two to three times as much as those in their middle age. There is therefore an incentive not only for governments but also for health insurance companies (who bear the financial load of supporting this age group) to improve health and decrease utilisation of services.

Large-scale health promotion programs were criticised in the early days for not causing reductions in heart disease death rates (McCormick & Skrabanek 1988). This led to the assumption that such interventions were unsuccessful. However, analysis of the data from a number of these programs shows that although mortality was not affected, there was a significant 'compression of morbidity' in older people, resulting in less need for health services in the later years. Fries, Green and Levine (1989) claim that, if quality of life is improved in the later years, active life expectancy—that is, those years in which disease is relatively absent—is extended. Hence, whereas people might not live any longer, they could 'die younger at an old age'. Evidence supporting this contention is emerging from research indicating that high-intensity strength training exercises are an effective and feasible means of preserving bone density while improving muscle mass, strength and balance in older people (Hunter et al. 2004).

This information is useful for developing policy that aims health promotion services at older adults.

Case study 8.6

Lessons learned from the tobacco experience for obesity control

The fight against smoking, which began with evidence of the adverse effects of smoking in the 1950s and was translated in earnest into anti-smoking programs in the early 1970s, has provided a number of lessons in changing population health. There are similar social, psychological and environmental factors between this and the modern obesity epidemic, which suggests that the key elements of an obesity control program should be (1) clinical intervention and management, with physicians being an effective way of doing so; (2) educational strategies, both at the individual and the population levels; (3) regulatory efforts, such as control of food outlets in vulnerable areas, such as schools; (4) economic approaches, through taxing and incentive schemes; and (5) the combination of all of these into comprehensive programs that address multiple facets of the environment simultaneously.

Mercer et al. 2003

Popular and unpopular health promotion

Health promotion, like any field of endeavour, can be positive or negative, depending on the way it is used. If education is simply a process of transferring allegiance from one activity to another—without thought for the reasons for doing so—the process of education might itself be in question. Similarly if health promotion results in a group of professionals deciding what is best, and setting out to program the population to behave in that way, the costs of such activity are likely to outweigh the benefits in the long run.

A second danger of overzealousness in the health field is the creation of increased anxiety and decreased pleasure of life. For example increased interest in health in some parts of the Western world has reached new heights. However, this has produced a subproportion of the population who could be classified as the 'worried well'; that is, although being perfectly healthy, their anxiety about the potential for being unwell drives them to use health services as much as (or more than) those who are actually unwell.

Popular health promotion also does little for those in real need. According to Worden (1979), bad health promotion is 'doing neat things with neat people' (see also Kok 1993). Consciousness raising, assertiveness training and up-market aerobics in the middle-class affluent population are all activities that have a role in setting a public stage for demand in health promotion services—but are they where the health promotion practitioners should be devoting their time and energy? Market forces tend to dominate these processes and might be left to work themselves out with little intervention on behalf of the practitioner. Market forces have little effect on programs for those who are in real need but do not have the ability to pay. Nevertheless, achieving changes for those in real need comes with its own set of frustrations for workers dedicated enough to struggle against the seemingly insurmountable structural barriers to good health in our society.

For health promotion practitioners pondering this dilemma, Syme (1997) offers some salient words of advice:

> I am convinced that insisting only on fundamental and revolutionary social change is dooming us to programs that will take years and generations to take effect. Since it is so difficult to implement such major changes, it is easy to ignore inequalities because, they say, nothing can realistically be done about them. Moral outrage about inequalities is appropriate but it may also be self-indulgent. If we really want to change the world we may have to begin in more modest but practical ways.

In chapters 9 and 10 we combine all of the information from the preceding chapters to look at a process for planning health promotion interventions and some useful skills and tools for the practitioner.

Note

1 For a detailed discussion of how these changes develop see *The Tipping Point* by Malcolm Gladwell (Back Bay Books, New York, 2002).

References

Bastion, H., 2002, 'Promoting drugs through hairdressers: is nothing sacred?', *Brit Med J* 325:1180.

Egger, G., 1991, 'Sports injuries in Australia: causes, costs and prevention', *Health Prom J Aust* 1(2):28–33.

Egger, G., Donovan, R., Giles-Corti, B., Bull, F., & Swinburn, B., 2001, 'Developing national physical activity guidelines for Australians', *Australian and New Zealand Journal of Public Health* 25(6):561–3.

Egger, G., Spark, R., & Donovan, R. A., 1990, 'Component circuit analysis to needs assessment and strategy selection in health promotion', *Health Prom Int* 5(4):299–302.

Fichtenberg, C. M., & Glantz, S. A., 2000, 'Association of the California Tobaccco Control Program with declines in cigarette consumption and mortality from heart disease', *New Eng J Med* 343(24):1772–7.

Fries, J. F., Green, L. W., & Levine, S., 1989, 'Health promotion and the compression of morbidity', *Lancet* March:481–3.

Green, L. W., & Kreuter, M. W., 1999, *Health Promotion Planning: An Educational and Environmental Approach*, Mayfield Publishing Co., Mountain View, Calif.

Green, L. W., & McAlister, A. L., 1984, 'Macro-intervention to support health behaviour: some theoretical perspectives and practical reflections', *Health Ed Quart* 11(3):332–9.

Hawe, P., Degeling, D., & Hall, J., 1990, *Evaluating Health Promotion: A Health Worker's Guide*, MacLennan & Petty, Sydney.

Hawe, P., Noort, M., King, L., & Jordens, C., 1997, 'Multiplying health gains: the critical role of capacity-building within health promotion programs', *Health Policy* 39:29–42.

Hawe, P., & Sheil, A., 1995, 'Preserving innovation under increasing accountability pressures: the health promotion investment portfolio approach', *Health Prom J Aust* 5(2):4–9.

Hunter, G. R., McCarthy, J. P., & Bamman, M. M., 2004, 'Effects of resistance training on older adults', *Sports Med* 34(5):329–48.

James, J., Thomas, P., Cavan, D., & Kerr, D., 2004, 'Preventing childhood obesity by reducing consumption of carbonated drinks: cluster randomised controlled trial', *Brit Med J* 328:1237–9.

Knowler, W. C., Barrett-Connor, E., Fowler, S. E., Hamman, R. F., Lachan, J. M., Walker, E. A., & Nathan, D. M., 2002, Diabetes Prevention Research Group. 'Reduction in the incidence of type 2 diabetes with lifestyle intervention or metformin', *N Engl J Med* 346:393–403.

Kok, G., 1993, 'Why are so many health promotion programs ineffective?', *Health Prom J Aust* 3(2):12–17.

Kotte, T., Batista, R., Defreise, G. & Brekke, M., 1988, 'Clinical trials of patient education for chronic conditions: a comparative meta analysis', *Prev Med* 259:2888–9.

Larson, E. B., Bergman, J., Heidrich, F., Alvin, B. L., & Schneeweiss, R., 1982, 'Do postcards improve influenza vaccination compliance?', *Med Care* 20:639–48.

Lasater, T. M., Carleton, R. A., & LeFebvre, R. C., 1988, 'The Pawtucket Heart Health Programme: utilising community resources for primary prevention', *Rhode Island Med J* 71:63–7.

Levine, D. M., Green, L. W., Deeds, S. G., Chwalow, J., Russell, R. P., & Finlay, J., 1979, 'Behavioural and clinical effects in randomised trials of health education with hypertensive patients', *J Am Med Assoc* 241(16):1700–3.

Lindstrom, J., Louheranta, A., Mannelin, M., Rastas, M., Salminen, V., Eriksson, J., Uusitupa, M., & Tuomilehto, J., 2003, Finnish Diabetes Prevention Study Group. 'The Finnish Diabetes Prevention Study (DPS): lifestyle intervention and 3-year results on diet and physical activity', *Diabetes Care* 26(12):3230–6.

Maiman, L. A., Green, L. W., Gibson, G., & Mackenzie, E. J., 1979, 'Education for self-treatment by adult asthmatics', *J Am Med Assoc* 241(18):1919–22.

McCormick, J., & Skrabanek, P., 1988, 'Coronary heart disease is not preventable by population interventions', *Lancet* 2:839–41.

McDermott, R., Tulip, F., Schmidt, B., & Sinha, A., 2001, 'Sustaining better diabetes care in remote indigenous Australian communities', *Brit Med J* 327:428–30.

Mercer, S. L., Green, L. W., Rosenthal, A. C., Husten, C. G., Khan, L. K., & Dietz, W. H., 2003, 'Possible lessons from the tobacco experience for obesity control', *Am J Clin Nutr* 77(4 Suppl):1073S–1082S.

NH&MRC (National Health & Medical Research Council), 1996, 'Promoting the health of Australians: case studies of achievements in improving the health of the population', AGPS, Pub. No. 2090, Canberra.

Puska, P., Toumilehto, J., & Salonen, J., 1981, *The North Karelia Projects: Evaluation of a Comprehensive Community Program for Control of Cardiovascular Disease in 1972–7 in North Karelia, Finland*, Public Health in Europe, WHO/EURO Monograph Series, Geneva.

Redman, S., Spencer, E., & Sanson-Fisher, R., 1990, 'The role of the mass media in changing health-related behaviour: a critical appraisal of two models', *Health Prom Int* 5(1):80–101.

Rentmeester, K. L., 1984, 'The economics of wellness promotion', *Prev Med* 9:6–9.

Rogerson, R. J., 1995, 'Environmental and health-related quality of life: conceptual and methodological similarities', *Soc Sci Med* 41(1):1373–82.

Russell, L. B., 1986, *Is Prevention Better Than Cure?*, Brookings Institution, Washington DC.

Spark, R., & Mills, P., 1988, 'Promoting Aboriginal health on television in the Northern Territory: a bicultural approach', *Drug Ed J Aust* 2(3):191–8.

Syme, L. S., 1997, 'Individual vs community interventions in public health practice: some thoughts about a new approach', *Health Promotion Matters* (VicHealth), 2:2–9.

Uusitupa, M., Lindi, V., Louheranta, A., Salopuro, T., Lindstrom, J., & Tuomilehto, J., 2003, 'Long-term improvement in insulin sensitivity by changing lifestyles of people with impaired glucose tolerance: four-year results from the Finnish diabetes prevention study', *Diabetes* 52(1):2532–8.

Worden, M., 1979, 'Popular and unpopular prevention', *J Drug Issues* Summer:425–32.

Chapter 9
Putting it all together: planning and developing health promotion initiatives

Summary of main points

- There are a number of different planning models for implementing health promotion.
- The tested PRECEDE–PROCEED model identifies key factors in any program and helps structure a program from the outset.
- Transition models such as SOPIE or COMBI can then provide a graduated, phased approach to putting a program into action.
- All appropriate approaches involve planning, implementation and evaluation.
- The selection of approaches is dependent on a number of factors, including the skills and preferences of the health promotion specialist and the desires of the target community.

Designing programs

In this chapter we attempt to bring together the practical aspects of designing an integrated health promotion program as discussed in the preceding chapters. This involves applying general principles of planning to the identification of needs and the development of strategies and methods to meet these needs. The development of a planned approach will depend on a range of factors, such as the nature of the topic to be addressed, the size of the intended audience, involvement of local authorities, the skills and operational preferences of the health promotion specialist and the desires of the target community. Planning a pool fencing campaign for a local government area in a New Zealand city, for example, would require a different perspective from planning an obesity reduction campaign for a Pacific Island country. Similarly, a plan to improve the nutrition of Indigenous people would require a different conceptualisation from a program to increase activity levels in a middle-class urban community.

Clearly, it would be nice to have a format for health promotion that could be applied on a formulaic basis, such as the 'best practice' system that is used in clinical medicine. However, as Green (2001) points out, best practice in medicine is relatively easy to determine, because it applies with some consistency to the relatively homogeneous physiology of the human species. Health promotion, on the other hand, deals with health behaviour, 'where social, cultural, economic, and other heterogeneities make the generalisability of any research more suspect'. According to Green, health promotion and other applications of health behavioural research thus need to replace 'best practices' with 'best processes'.

A number of planning models have been described,[1] all of which have value under certain circumstances. Some are based on strategies for different phases of the lifespan (Edelman et al. 2002; Murray & Zentnor 2000); others are specifically settings-based, such as within workplaces (i.e. Cox 2003), or in clinical practice (Woolf, Jonas & Lawrence 1996). Perhaps the simplest distillation applicable to most situations is that shown in figure 9.1, which has been modified from one of the most widely accepted exponents in this area (Green & Kreuter 1999).

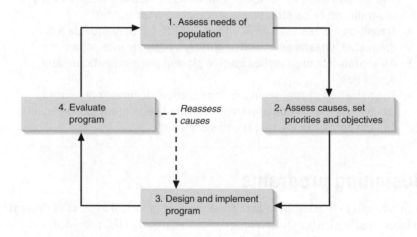

Figure 9.1: Green's basic steps in program planning and implementation
Green & Kreuter 1999

In this model, phase 1 implies an epidemiological approach to identifying populations at risk and determining needs. This can be done in a structured fashion using such techniques as the component circuit approach described in chapter 8. In phase 2, risk factors are identified, both behavioural (e.g. alcohol, tobacco, physical inactivity, diet, unsafe driving behaviour) and structural (e.g. poor housing, unemployment, unsafe work environments), along with Green's (Green & Kreuter 1999) predisposing, enabling and reinforcing factors (see below). Phase 3 involves the design and implementation of a program to deal with this, and phase 4 looks at evaluation and either reassessment or continuation of the program (Green & Kreuter 1999).

PRECEDE–PROCEED

Part of this approach involves the widely used PRECEDE–PROCEED model of Green and Kreuter (1999), which is probably the most widely used planning model in the health promotion literature, and in practice.

The model is shown in figure 9.2. The value of Green's model (which has undergone a number of modifications since first presented as just PRECEDE) is that it makes clear that the factors analysed in the planning and development phases (the PRECEDE phases) are the same factors to be considered in the implementation and evaluation phases (PROCEED).

PRECEDE is an acronym for Predisposing, Reinforcing and Enabling Constructs in Educational (and Environmental) Diagnosis and Evaluation. The novelty of this framework is that it focuses on outcomes rather than inputs, forcing the health practitioner to begin the planning process from the outcome end. It is also comprehensive in that each of the five phases in PRECEDE defines a different layer of diagnosis: social, epidemiological, behavioural, educational and administrative.

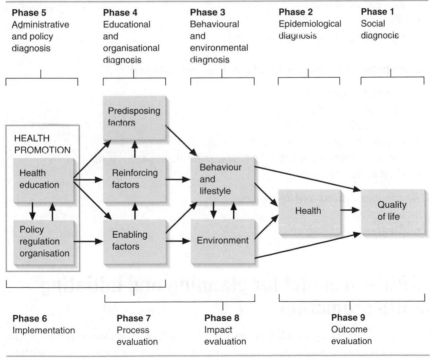

Figure 9.2: The PRECEDE–PROCEED model for health promotion planning and evaluation
Green & Kreuter 1999

Green's model was later expanded to include a more environmental orientation to health problems by including PROCEED: an acronym for Policy, Regulatory and Organisational Constructs in Educational and Environmental Development. PROCEED includes resource mobilisation and evaluation, and is essentially an elaboration and extension of the administrative diagnostic phase of PRECEDE. Overall, the addition of PROCEED to the original model gave greater emphasis to the contribution of structural factors and community organisation processes to program implementation.

Case study 9.1

A sample concept brief for planning

An example of a concept brief to help health promotion practitioners and funding authorities plan health promotion initiatives should include the following headings:

Scope
- Project description
- Key deliverables
- Rationale
- Reach (e.g. local, state, national)

Preliminary key partner/stakeholder interest/support

Indicative project costs
- Permanent staff
- Consumables
- Project budget
- Level of confidence in cost estimates (low, medium, high)
- Cost implications

Recommendations and decisions
- Next step
- Clearances and so on.

SOPIE—a model for planning and initiating health promotion

A slightly different approach to planning, but one that incorporates all of the above, is a planning model using the acronym SOPIE, which the current authors have previously used for planning social marketing campaigns (Egger, Donovan & Spark 1993). The stages are just as relevant for planning health promotion programs in general. They are:

- Situational analysis
- Objective setting
- Planning
- Implementation
- Evaluation.

The SOPIE approach has been used in Pacific Island countries to help structure interventions aimed at reducing chronic non-communicable diseases, such as diabetes and obesity, as well as in smaller-scale social experiments, such as in encouraging older people to eat more fibre (see case study 6.3). The background of this approach indicates its bias towards a social marketing or community organisational approach to health promotion; however, the process and stages are not exclusive of other, if not all, large-scale health promotion initiatives. The stages of the process are shown below. Each stage is then discussed in detail.

The SOPIE model for health promotion interventions

The stages of the SOPIE model, defined by the acronym, are summarised below. A summary of the processes within each stage is given.

- **Situational analysis**: identifying the issue, specifying the problem, identifying potential target audiences and strategies, assessing resources, formative research.
- **Objective setting**: defining overall goals and campaign goals, specific behavioural and communication objectives for the target audiences.
- **Planning**: devising message strategies, developing and pre-testing materials, selecting media, identifying supporting components.
- **Implementation**: developing detailed program procedures, involving other sectors and stakeholders, program management.
- **Evaluation**: campaign monitoring, process and outcome evaluation.
- **Analysing**: the problem, the market, the potential strategies.

Stage 1: Situational analysis

This stage is intended to identify and accurately represent the extent of the problem or issue and to identify possible causes. It is perhaps the most important stage of any campaign and that for which most input is necessary. There are four distinct phases within this stage:

1. Identifying the problem

Problem identification can come from a number of sources, including the media, literature reviews, epidemiological data, political interest, statistics, needs analysis (see chapter 8) or public pressure. Data representing the problem is also helpful in selling the program. A further and important part of this stage is in determining the propitiousness of an intervention at any particular time. Although there might be a need because of the frequency and severity of the problem, social (and political) attitudes can influence the process of priority setting. Public acceptance of both the problem and the solution is thus an important ingredient for successful intervention. The practical elements of analysis therefore include:

1. the nature and extent of the problem (e.g. frequency, severity and so on)
2. the level of evidence relating to the proposed problem (e.g. will decreasing smoking consumption actually reduce lung cancer?)
3. public and political acceptance for (a) an action to be taken and (b) the proposed action to be taken (e.g. would the public accept, and would politicians pay for, a major campaign that persuaded people to quit smoking?).

It should be noted that often the problem is not as it initially seems. Early campaigns aimed at reducing smoking, for example, were based on increasing knowledge of the health risks of smoking. As these results became known, it was clearer that the problem was not so much knowledge but feelings of being able to quit and bending to social pressure to quit. Problem identification at this stage showed that programs emphasising the socially unacceptable aspects of smoking, in an environment that tolerated and even facilitated smoking, were likely to be more successful.

2. Defining the intended audience

Once a problem is identified, there is a need for a clear idea of the intended audience (see chapter 5). The intended audience is not necessarily those among whom the problem is greatest. It might be those who are most likely to be influenced, given the available resources; that is, where the biggest 'bang for the buck' lies.

Smokers, for example, can be segmented according to a number of factors: age, sex, length of time smoking, acceptance of health messages or willingness to quit. A segment selected for a quit smoking message, however, might not necessarily be the largest (e.g. young women) but could be smokers with the most to gain or those who are the easiest to reach, given limited resources. A different approach might be necessary for different audiences.

3. Identifying possible strategies

In this stage of planning, the viability of using different strategies as outlined throughout this text is assessed, and the role each is to play *vis-à-vis* other strategies is determined. Furthermore, any comprehensive program must consider and select all strategies that can add to the aims of the program. This

Case study 9.2

COMBI—a strategic planning model from the World Health Organization

There are many planning models that can be used for health promotion. COMBI (Communication for Behavioural Impact) is one of these designed to help plan, implement and monitor a variety of communication actions. COMBI has been developed by WHO and applied to a number of health issues in developing countries, including dengue fever prevention and control and other communicable disease applications. As a social mobilisation and communication model, COMBI is equally relevant to non-communicable or chronic diseases. There are three phases in the model: planning, implementation and monitoring, and evaluation. The planning phase consists of fifteen steps, as shown below:

1. assemble a multidisciplinary planning team
2. state preliminary behavioural objectives
3. plan and conduct formative research
4. invite feedback on formative research
5. analyse, prioritise and specify final desired behavioural outcomes
6. segment target groups
7. develop your strategy
8. pre-test behaviour, messages and materials
9. establish a monitoring system
10. strengthen staff skills
11. set up a system to manage and share information
12. structure your program
13. write a strategic implementation plan
14. determine your budget
15. conduct a pilot test and revise your strategic plan.

Each of the other phases also provides a detailed 'road-map' to follow in designing a health promotion program.

Parks & Lloyd 2004
Also see www.who.infectious-disease-report/2002/behaviour.html and
www.comminit.com/pdf/Combi4-pager_Nov_14.pdf

could include changes in availability of products or materials (e.g. higher taxes on energy-dense foods that lead to obesity, restriction of fast-food outlets and so on) and changes in conditions that encourage over-eating (e.g. improvements in school canteens), as well as capacity building to help progression towards an end goal. As suggested by the epidemiological triad considered in chapter 1, it is only when all corners of the triad are considered that an epidemic can be truly managed.

4. Generating a strategic concept

Where appropriate, ideas for a project concept or major theme are often developed at this stage using either formative research or skilled assessment by health professionals. A strategic concept is a broad approach to the issue at hand that provides direction for the definition of communication objectives and the development of program strategies. For instance, in the case of skin cancer prevention, a concept might be to encourage greater use of shaded environments. This might then lead on to a strategy of either working with local communities and authorities to provide more shade or developing a media campaign to encourage individuals to seek existing shade options. In the latter instance the concept would be developed fully into a social marketing message.

A summary of tasks and signposts in phase 1

Main tasks

- Get agreement and cooperation of local authorities to commence a project.
- Collect and analyse available local and regional statistics.
- Arrange meetings with health professionals and key stakeholders.
- Set up an audit of existing facilities and potential opportunities and establish feasibility of how to proceed. Includes planning for next steps.
- Begin to identify potential partner groups and key personnel within them.
- Discuss possibilities and needs for next phase (i.e. baseline capacity building, environmental diagnosis, baseline data collection etc.).

Key signposts

- Identification of one or more personnel to act as operational manager and/or advocates of any intervention initiative over the long term.
- Development of ownership by local community.
- Recognition of the problem and commitment to do something about this by key local authorities.
- Commitment of local officials to work with the health promotion team.
- Agreement of potential partners to become involved.
- Commitment by local connections to arrange workshops on later visits.

Stage 2: Objective setting

On the basis of the identified problem and the selection of intended audiences, the next step is to set overall goals and specific behavioural and communication objectives for the intended audience(s).

1. Defining goals

Goals help to determine the direction of an intervention and set forth what the program hopes to achieve. Goals are written as broad general statements. An example related to sexually transmitted diseases might be: 'to decrease infertility owing to STDs'.

Because they are broad and general, goals do not specify the method of intervention. Hence they need to be accompanied by measurable objectives.

2. Setting objectives

The planning stage of any project is designed to provide a blueprint for action. As part of this, there is a need for a set of clear-cut objectives to be determined with the local community. Ideally, the objectives of a well-planned campaign should be specific, time-related and measurable. They can be defined in terms of the ultimately desirable outcome (e.g. reduced morbidity) or intermediate objectives, such as target population knowledge, attitudes and behaviour; changes in the physical environment; or public policy or practices related to health. These are thus called 'outcome objectives'. In the case of motor vehicle injuries, outcome objectives of a preventive initiative might be reduced fatalities, but intermediate measures such as a reduction in driver blood alcohol levels, or even reduction of alcohol consumption in a targeted area, could also be included as outcome objectives.

Project objectives must be realistic. What can be achieved by one campaign of limited duration must not be confused with what it is hoped could be achieved by a series of campaigns and a combination of strategies that would be part of a long-term program.

3. Capacity building, stakeholder involvement and environmental diagnosis

This stage can include capacity building, particularly where it is likely to be important for later health-care worker involvement. In the case of type 2 diabetes prevention, for example, training in management of obesity and weight control for clinicians might be a vital component of any program. This can also help to ensure greater cooperation of medical and other health professionals in ongoing program development. Capacity building of health-care workers in the basic principles of health promotion (e.g. social marketing, community development) can also be included here.

Because any initiatives must be developed and 'owned' by the community in which they are to be enacted, key stakeholders need to be incorporated into any planning decisions. One way of doing so is by involving these people in an environmental analysis, such as using the ANGELO model (see chapter 8), which then serves the dual function of increasing community involvement as well as helping the community define its own issues.

A summary of tasks and signposts in stage 2

Main tasks

- Building community links.
- Baseline capacity building (e.g. education of medical and allied health professionals).
- Environmental diagnosis (e.g. ANGELO) and stakeholder involvement.
- Enhancing health promotion capacity (e.g. by workshops with local health promotion staff).
- Setting potential goals and objectives with health personnel.

Key signposts

- Increased basic skills among local health workers.
- Commitment of local health personnel and key stakeholders.
- Ordered priorities in environmental and other initiatives.
- Commencement of up-skilling of health promotion staff.
- Commitment to proceed to the next level.

Stage 3: Planning

Once detailed objectives have been set, the next step is to develop specific project components. The viability and affordability of different potential strategies needs to be assessed; message strategies and the media for their dissemination need to be identified; monitoring and evaluation procedures should be specified; pre-testing undertaken where necessary; and other back-up strategies devised. The role of other sectors needs to be defined and their cooperation sought. Adequate resources must be available to meet the anticipated response to the campaign (e.g. domestic violence campaigns also inevitably result in a large number of abused people seeking counselling).

Choosing the method

Once strategies have been devised, the methods of operation within them need to be considered. If awareness raising through social marketing is an option, different approaches to delivering the message should be considered. Mass media advertising is expensive but allows full control over message exposure and greater flexibility in presentation; publicity is relatively inexpensive but depends to a great extent on the 'newsworthiness' of a topic; edutainment is even less able to be controlled by the message initiator and is likely to work only over the long term. Choice of method also depends on the target audience, the project objectives and the budget, as well as the availability of appropriate skills to the health team.

Primary and secondary media should also be identified and, in the case of advertising, media schedules developed to provide optimal coverage. Where advocacy is the desired outcome, media should be identified for targeting to get the desired message across. The planning mix also involves consideration of the five Ms of promotion: the Market (target audience), the Message, the Media, the Method and the Measures (see Donovan & Henley 2003).

Where a community process is selected as an appropriate strategy, methods of involving the community such as through social mobilisation, leader or skill group meetings, or partnership arrangements might need to be considered.

Developing the message

Message development involves first getting the right message, and second getting the message right, to deliver it in a way that is likely to be most effective. Given a behavioural or attitudinal objective, developing a message strategy attempts to answer the question: what sort of motivations must be aroused or what sort of beliefs need to be established in the receiver's minds to bring about these behavioural or attitudinal changes? The primary tools for message strategy development (i.e. getting the right message) are qualitative research techniques, such as individual in-depth interviews and focus group discussions with members of the target audience.

The message strategy should include the following elements, although not always in every individual message execution:

1. the benefits promised by adopting the recommended behaviour or attitude (i.e. the motivational component)
2. specific actions that the individual or community can undertake, whether intermediate (e.g. call a hotline) or related to the desired end-behaviour
3. reassurances that the recommended course of action is efficacious
4. reassurances that the individual or community is capable of carrying out the recommended course of action (with appropriate assistance where relevant).

Where more than one strategy is used (e.g. social marketing and capacity building), which usually should be the case, the relative roles of the strategies and methods within them need to be established and the subsequent messages for each method developed with these different objectives in mind.

The project objective should serve as a reference for measuring the project outcome; for example if the objective is to decrease smoking to make people feel better, measures of wellbeing can be included in the campaign evaluation.

Testing the message

Before full-scale implementation of a project, messages should be pre-tested. This can include such processes as concept testing and efficacy testing (Donovan

& Henley 2003). Pre-testing messages at this stage can provide direction for improving the message or identifying which of several alternative strategies for execution has the greatest potential. Models are available for this stage of the planning including the guidebook *Pretesting in Health* produced by the US National Cancer Institute.

A summary of tasks and signposts in stage 3

Main tasks

- Planning for an ongoing and sustainable project.
- Linking of allied groups.
- Further education (e.g. of medical and health professionals) where appropriate.
- Consideration of evaluation methods and baseline evaluation research.
- Planning of an awareness-raising 'umbrella' where appropriate and possible.
- Development of health promotion ads and materials if this is appropriate.
- Selection of main messages and methods of delivery.

Key signposts

- Development of an ongoing and sustainable action plan.
- Development of an evaluation strategy.
- Consideration of awareness raising and community involvement strategies.
- Increased local skills in strategy implementation.

Stage 4: Implementation

Implementing a health promotion program includes setting process objectives (i.e. what is to be accomplished, by whom and when), managing the implementation process (i.e. coordination, intersectoral liaison and so on), monitoring the process and being prepared for any negative responses to the campaign.

'Process objectives' detail the level of activities designed to produce the desired outcomes. They describe the relationship between a project's activities and the desired outcomes. Process objectives are thus not simply lists of activities, but are quantifiable and measurable statements of what the project will have accomplished by certain dates. For reducing motor vehicle injuries, for example, process objectives would include the number of community service announcements to be aired by a certain date and the number of media releases to have been issued by that date, but also could include an awareness of what proportion of the target population was exposed to the message.

Some projects involve a staged 'roll-out' of strategies. The first stage of an anti-smoking implementation, for example, might concentrate on an increased knowledge of less well-known risks (e.g. passive smoking). The second and later stages might be advocacy, aimed at increasing pressure on workplace managers to avoid the risk of litigation from those affected by passive smoking, by banning smoking in certain areas of the workplace. Health promotion projects using the media in 'new' topic areas, about which knowledge and awareness is low, often aim initially at educating (or informing) about the problem, then run a second stage to motivate (or persuade) people to do something about it. Advocacy can then often add to the advantages achieved by increased awareness.

Monitoring is important in the implementation stage to ensure that appropriate changes are occurring and to evaluate the process of operation. This is often done through a recording of requests received about a program or other tracking measures. Enquiries for further information, increased demand for project materials or courses, or increases in the sales of appropriate products (e.g. fruits and vegetables, exercise equipment, nicotine chewing gum or increased gym memberships), for example, could be indirect measures of whether the message is reaching and influencing its target audience.

It should also be recognised that often vested interests will be opposed to project methods that seek to alter the status quo, and reaction from them is likely to come at the implementation stage of any campaign. Cigarette and alcohol manufacturers, for example, form a powerful lobby group against the introduction of campaigns designed to reduce smoking and drinking. The Sporting Shooters' Association is able to thwart most attempts at gun control advocacy, despite the fact that firearms are a major cause of intentional and unintentional homicide, and food and grocery manufacturers will try to counter any attempts to reduce the sale of certain foods and soft drinks.

If possible, these contingencies should be forecast in the planning stages and approaches developed for coping with them as they arise. In some cases, interference in a health promotion project has been used by health professionals to create publicity around a promotion, which ensures that it achieves a wider exposure than might otherwise have occurred. Anti-smoking groups like ASH (Action on Smoking and Health) are particularly skilful in creating publicity by raising the ire of tobacco companies.

In this phase, demand should be anticipated for the increased need for 'on-the-ground' services. A quit smoking project, for example, might increase the need for quit smoking courses, self-help groups and nicotine patches and gums; diabetes prevention might stimulate an interest in weight control and exercise programs; and traffic injury prevention might require driver training skills. These needs should be anticipated in the early stage of the project to ensure adequate resource allocation and the continuation of momentum of the project once it has begun.

A summary of tasks and signposts in stage 4

Main tasks

- Putting the plan into action.
- Involving all selected strategies and methods and community involvement in them.
- Establishing 'on-the-ground' services (e.g. quit smoking groups, weight loss education centres etc.); ongoing capacity building of health professionals.
- Developing advocacy skills.

Key signposts

- Acceptance of a program by local media and policy makers in the community.
- Social marketing media being aired (if appropriate).
- Advocacy taken up by media and other outlets.
- Commencement of community approaches such as community-based group or NGO involvement.
- Establishment of work practice outlines among health promotion staff.

Stage 5: Evaluation

Evaluation involves a systematic assessment of the degree to which an intervention is meeting its objectives. If the budget allows, it should be carried out midway through a campaign to correct any deficiencies or capitalise on any new opportunities that present themselves, as well as at the end of the program. Methods of carrying out process, impact and outcome evaluation are dealt with in other publications (Rootman et al. 2000; Valente 2002).

In general, evaluation measures should be in place before a program is initiated. However, in some circumstances, changes in events as a result of the intervention could lead to a modification of the program. If monitoring shows a disappointing response to the project messages, for example, there might be a need to institute measures to find out why this is so. The lack of response by smokers to a 'Quit and Win' campaign in New South Wales, which offered the possibility of winning a car, led to the need for some quick focus groups with smokers to refocus the campaign midway through a paid media schedule (Chapman et al. 1993). The focus groups showed that although the competition was well received by non-smoking family and friends of smokers, smokers felt besieged by anti-smoking warnings and pressures. Although desperately wanting to quit, many had tried and failed and did not wish to be reminded of the fact—even given the (albeit slim) possibility of winning a car. The message therefore needed to be changed to involve more smokers' non-smoking contacts.

Evaluation is often thought of as a luxury in health promotion campaigns where the political imperative is simply to be seen to be doing something for the good of the electorate. Funding for evaluation is often not included in budgets allocated by those who don't appreciate the importance of evaluation. However, it is often these same funding sources (e.g. politicians) who use evaluation results to either confirm or deny the value of their funding allocations when they are put under scrutiny. Funding for evaluation should be seen as an integral part of any health promotion program. A rule of thumb for this allocation would be approximately 10 per cent of the total health promotion budget.

A summary of tasks and signposts in stage 5

Main tasks

- Identification and establishment of 'process' goals (e.g. increases in awareness, knowledge, receipt of messages, involvement in appropriate actions, improved skills, environmental change etc.).
- Identification and establishment of outcome evaluation (e.g. using existing databases or carrying out pre- and post-test sampling of BMI, waist circumference etc.).
- Statistical analysis of results.
- Ongoing assistance and advice.
- Report writing.

Key signposts

- Collection of evaluation data.
- Written report.
- Comparison of outcomes with initial objectives.
- Documented forward planning with local staff.

Summary

Health promotion initiatives are generally presented in the form of ongoing projects or 'interventions'. This requires a knowledge of factors such as those expanded in Green and Kreuter's PRECEDE–PROCEED model, as well as a graduated process of conducting such a project. The SOPIE model is one such process for putting all the skills and tools discussed throughout this text into practice towards the goal of better health and improved quality of life for all. There are, however, a number of other models, and the selection of them will depend on a number of factors, including the demands of the community and the skills and preferences of the health promotion practitioner.

Note

1 For a summary of a number of communication models see www. comminit.com/planning_models.html

References

Chapman, S., Smith, W., Mowbray, G., & Egger, G., 1993, ' "Quit and Win" smoking cessation contests: how should effectiveness be evaluated?', *Prev Med* 22(3):423–32.

Cox, C. C., 2003, *ACSMs Worksite Health Promotion Manual: A Guide to Building and Sustaining Healthy Worksites*, Human Kinetics Publishers, Champaign, Ill.

Donovan, R. J., & Henley, N., 2003, *Social Marketing: Principles and Practice*, IP Communications, Melbourne, Vic.

Edelman, C., Mandel, C. L., & Edelman, C. L., 2002, *Health Promotion Throughout the Lifespan* (5th edn), C. V. Mosby, St Louis.

Egger, G., Donovan, R., & Spark, R., 1993, *Health and the Media*, McGraw-Hill, Sydney.

Green, L. W., 2001, 'From research to "best practices" in other settings and populations', *Am J Health Behav* 25(3):165–78.

Green, L. W., & Kreuter, M., 1999, *Health Promotion Planning: An Educational and Ecological Approach* (3rd edn), Mayfield, Toronto.

Murray, R. B., & Zentner, J. P., 2000, *Health Promotion Strategies Throughout the Lifespan* (7th edn), Prentice Hall, Upper Saddle River, NJ.

National Cancer Institute, 1982, *Pretesting in Health*, National Cancer Institute Report, New York.

Parks, W., & Lloyd, L., 2004, *Planning Social Mobilisation and Communication for Dengue Fever Prevention and Control: A Step-by-Step Guide*, WHO, Geneva.

Rootman, I., Goodstaff, M., Hyndman, B., McQueen, D. V., Potvin, L., Spingett, J., & Ziglio, E., 2000, *Evaluating Health Promotion: Principles and Perspectives*, WHO Regional Publications (European Series), WHO, Geneva.

Valente, T. W., 2002, *Evaluating Health Promotion Programs*, Oxford University Press, Oxford.

Woolf, S. H., Jonas, S., & Lawrence, R. S., 1996, *Health Promotion and Disease Prevention in Clinical Practice*, Lippincott, Williams & Wilkins, New York.

Chapter 10
Skills, tools and competencies for health promotion

Summary of main points

- 'Skills' are defined as the ability to facilitate a particular process successfully. Tools are a means of doing so through available techniques.
- Health promotion practitioners need skills and tools that cross the boundaries of many other professions.
- The wider the health promotion practitioner's repertoire of skills, the greater the options available for dealing with any issue.
- Although content knowledge is important, process skills differentiate the health promotion practitioner from other health professionals.
- Skills range from writing, community facilitation and political acumen, to clinical, evaluation and social marketing ability. Tools include presentation, diagnosis and capacity building processes.
- The competencies required for health promotion are specified in professional standards documents.

The need for specialist skills

As an art/science, health promotion requires a unique range of skills and operational tools that cross the boundaries of several other professions. At one extreme, there are advantages in having clinical skills for dealing with patients or clients on a one-to-one basis, whether as a medical practitioner or an allied health professional. At the other extreme, there are the political, lobbying and social advocacy skills that can help set the agenda for changes at the population level. Within each of these areas there are established tools, such as clinical methods, communication skills, screening tests and educational approaches for enabling the process of health promotion to occur. Not all are likely to be within the repertoire of a single health promotional practitioner. However, the wider the repertoire, the greater the options available for dealing with any particular issue. Developing applied skills and ability to use tools also widens the opportunity for employment for health promotion practitioners outside the health sector, such as in community work, advertising, market research, media, journalism or public policy, should this become desired or necessary.

In contrast to the content of health issues, which involves some basic biological, psychological and epidemiological knowledge, skills and tools facilitate the process of health promotion. As with this text in general, some level of health science content is assumed. A range of process skills and tools for disseminating this content and implementing health promotion initiatives for an intended audience is outlined below. This is not definitive and will need to be added to, as new tools become available. 'Skills' are defined as the ability to facilitate a particular process successfully. Tools are a means of doing so through available techniques. It is these that differentiate the health promotion practitioner from other health professionals. In the final part of this chapter we list a number of competencies regarded as desirable for health promotion practitioners under the headings described in the SOPIE model discussed in chapter 9.

Skills for health promotion

The following is a list of essential skills for health promotion professionals:

- *Organisation and planning ability.* Any health promotion intervention requires detailed organisation and planning and the ability to work in concert with locally identified personnel.
- *Interviewing and listening skills.* Much formative work in the early stages of any project requires the ability to interview key stakeholders and interpret the results of the interviews for functional interventions. Communication and an ability to develop empathy with a variety of different people, which could include Indigenous, minority, and culturally and linguistically diverse (CALD) groups, is also vital.
- *Teaching ability.* This is required at different levels to increase background knowledge among professionals, stakeholders and community members, and could include didactic lecturing, interactive learning processes or education through a range of different media.
- *Group facilitation.* The ability to organise and run small groups and understand group dynamics is essential for a number of processes in health promotion, including those listed above.
- *Media skills.* This includes the basics of transmitting health messages through the select use of appropriate media channels. The ability to use all mass media and limited media avenues available in the theatre of operation is a necessary prerequisite for successful health promotion.

Case study 10.1

The legacy of Sir Richard Doll

Recognised as the father of modern epidemiology, British doctor Sir Richard Doll was the first to recognise the link between smoking and disease in the early 1950s when he noticed differences in death rates between smoking and non-smoking doctors. Over the next half century, Doll's work has been credited with turning the tide against smoking and providing a model for health promotion. Still publishing at the age of 100, Sir Richard was able to confirm his earlier data in a fifty-year follow-up of British doctors in 2001, which proved that men who smoked, and continued to smoke, died on average about ten years younger than lifelong non-smokers. Cessation at the ages of 60, 50, 40, or 30 gained respectively about 3, 6, 9, or 10 years of life expectancy. Death rates at all ages beyond 35 were shown to be two to three times higher among smokers than non-smokers. However, quitting at the age of 30 can help smokers avoid almost all the risk of early death.

Doll et al. 2004

- *Collaboration.* The ability to work collaboratively with a range of different disciplines, including:
  - graphic artists and creative personnel
  - statisticians
  - medical professionals
  - academics and researchers.
- *Report writing ability.* Writing at the academic level is necessary to pass on information about successes and failures achieved within any program. All interventions should be conducted with a view to academic publication. This includes the ability to successfully 'translate' scientific evidence into understandable language.
- *Evaluation skills.* The ability to evaluate a project at any of a number of levels is vital if a health promotion project is to receive ongoing support.
- *Political skills.* 'Political' is meant here in the broad sense of understanding interactions between professionals, stakeholders and the community in general, particularly where these interactions might be able to influence healthy public policy.
- *Ability to source and understand evidence-based content material.* Although not everything about a health issue needs to be understood to communicate key aspects of it, it is important for health promotion professionals to know how to access the scientific literature to confirm areas of possible controversy and understand the evidence base. In recent times this involves knowledge of Internet searching techniques and an understanding of levels of acceptance of scientific evidence.

Additional skills

Additional desirable skills include:

- *Ability to facilitate community development/organisational processes.* The process of working in different sized communities and enabling them to develop mechanisms for health promotion from within is a vital component of many health promotion interventions.
- *Clinical (one-on-one) lifestyle counselling.* This represents the grassroots of health promotion, which is often overlooked by many non-clinical professionals. However, it is a useful skill for anyone likely to be involved in facilitating behaviour change.
- *Social marketing skills.* Social marketing is an element of most modern health promotion interventions, particularly those requiring widespread population knowledge change and awareness. The skills required within social marketing include:

  (a) *Ability to conduct formative research (e.g. focus groups).* Focus group (qualitative) research can help form an understanding of any intervention to follow and provide ideas about the content of these promotions.

  (b) *Ability to train community participants in formative research techniques.* This involves conducting training programs incorporating community groups with feedback from facilitators and information from community groups.

  (c) *Ability to write and oversee scripts for TV and radio ads.* The electronic media are particularly effective for awareness raising and agenda setting. Ability to write and supervise the making of health promotion messages is a useful asset in these situations.

  (d) *Ability to prepare a creative brief.* Where sophisticated media messages are required and professional communicators such as advertising or public relations personnel are used, a brief providing scientific background and limitations and directions for messages is often needed from a health professional.

  (e) *Identifying target audiences.* The identification of target groups through various techniques allows a more focused approach and greater likelihood of an effective media spread.

  (f) *Advocacy skills.* Effective use of appropriate media is vital to health promotion. Advocacy is one way of doing so through the media.

- *Survey and sampling knowledge.* Although health promotion professionals themselves might not require such knowledge, an awareness of the appropriate techniques enables a more effective supervision of planning and evaluation research.
- *'Train the trainer' skills.* Much health promotion involves working directly with health professionals to expand content knowledge in such areas as infectious diseases, physical fitness, nutrition, weight control,

stress management, drug abuse and so on. Ability to build capacity through trainer training is a useful skill.

Some principles for working in disadvantaged communities and developing countries

There are a number of principles involved in health promotion activities that, although often not defined, are standard throughout developing countries and disadvantaged communities. The list outlined below has been developed from personal experience of the authors in this capacity:

- **Things do not happen quickly**. Health behaviour change is a slow process, which requires first awareness, then agreement, then consensus of the key stakeholders involved.
- **Plan ahead**. Time is always best spent in a country or community if it is well planned in advance. If not living in that community, this might be only minimally possible on a first visit; however, key contacts should be made beforehand and meetings arranged as they see fit.
- **Find a local advocate to manage the process**. If there is to be success, it will depend on one or a small number of enthusiastic advocates who can help drive the program from within. Such a person might or might not come from the health sector, but could also be a key mover from the general community. They should be used as a vital resource and provided with the best possible information and training.
- **Devolve to the community**. Any program will only ever be as successful as the people in the home community who drive it on an ongoing basis. Long-term health change requires continuous input, and outside assistants cannot and should not be expected to provide it on an ongoing basis. The program must belong to the community with the assistant being merely a catalyst.
- **Be flexible**. As a result of the gradual process of change it is not always possible for plans to be met. If this causes frustration, the community can see it as a lack of understanding, and this can result in alienation, which is very difficult to reverse.
- **Expect down times**. These are inevitable and could result from changes in plans or failure of meetings to materialise, to whole visits that might be less productive than initially planned. Weather (particularly during monsoon seasons) is sometimes a limiting factor in developing countries in the Asia–Pacific region, and this might be a consideration in planning short-term projects.
- **Get into the culture**. First visits to a new community or country will always involve a fast learning curve when it is necessary to learn

cultural practices and mores. This should involve fraternisation to the extent that it is permitted in the community. Developing good social ties is likely to engender trust for future ongoing relationships.

- **Develop rapport**. As with any one-on-one clinical relationship, no behaviour change is likely to occur until trust and rapport is developed with the client (in this case the community). This will take time, and hence the early stages of any program should be spent nurturing this relationship with all aspects of the population (e.g. the media, stakeholders, health sector personnel).

- **Work within the existing frameworks**. As early as possible in a program, time should be spent in consultation with those in the health service who are likely to have the most influence. This is often not just the local doctors but also nurses and other health workers.

- **Work with, not alongside or against, local structures**. Religion forms a large part of life in many developing countries, but in some cases (e.g. the Pacific) it also plays an unwitting role in the facilitation of certain potentially unhealthy practices, such as feasting and inactivity. On the other hand, church leaders can be major instigators of change if they are advised of the health problems these practices can create for their communities. Church leaders can also become key advocates for health promotion.

- **Select local advocates on the basis of enthusiasm and commitment**. Although it is important to have a sound base of knowledge relating to the content area of health being considered, local advocates can readily acquire the necessary amount of it provided they are enthusiastic and passionate about making a difference in their community and have the will to remain committed over the long haul.

- **Don't automatically assume that what works in one country or community will work in another**. A basic principle in designing health promotion interventions is the three words 'it all depends'. This means that interventions must be specific and dependent on a range of conditions.

- **Don't forget the impact of any initiatives on funding sources**. Although sources of funding should not dictate the direction of a health promotion program, visible actions that get early 'runs on the board' (e.g. such as in social marketing or the media) can build momentum among policy makers for future funding for sustainability of any project.

- **Know your boundaries**. Most cultures have several layers, some of which are available to the visitor, but others are kept personal and even undisclosed. Not only is it a mistake to think that they could be breached by an outsider but also it could be offensive to do so. Hence, although you might be invited to participate in certain activities in a community, you could lose favour by attempting to become involved in others.

- **As far as possible, check your opinions with others before making conclusions**. Working in different cultures often means coming to conclusions on the basis of one's own culture. By working with others in the field, ideas can be compared and conclusions checked before basing further actions on what could be a misconception.
- **Begin with humility**. Any intruder into a new area can find their input blocked by locals, or other consultant health workers, who might feel threatened by an over-aggressive approach. Until rapport is established, humility is imperative, combined with polite listening and questioning skills.
- **Always ask whether something should be done**. With tasks such as filming, conducting training, meeting stakeholders and so on, it is important to find out whether what you want to do is acceptable in that context. In some instances, status might prohibit the use of certain protocols, and ignoring this might mean permanent difficulty in further operations. If possible, develop a relationship with a trusted advocate who can advise on the appropriate behaviour.
- **Build local capacity**. Avoid being a 'parachute consultant' by maintaining relationships and support in the period following your visit (particularly if this is a short-term project).
- **Look for and be conscious of local power structures**. As in all cultures and communities, not everyone in a particular working environment gets along. If interpersonal interactions are not detected, barriers can be formed against future progress. It is important therefore not only to recognise allegiances but also to avoid becoming involved in them. (Difficulties often come from 'turf wars' with professional colleagues as much as or more than with locals.)
- **Carry out everything with a view to documentation for sustainability**. Although not all health promotion activities are publishable, it is important to keep scientific publication in mind as an end process of any potential action. Too often health promotion interventions, both successful and unsuccessful, are not reported, leaving future projects to reinvent the wheel. Although publishing is vital for future progress by those who follow, all of the above rules should be considered before attempting to publish.

Egger 2004

Tools for health promotion

Health promotion tools include aids to communication and education, diagnosis, capacity building and measurement. The list of these is long, varied and evolving, and might depend on the experience of the health promotion practitioner. Some of the main tools available include:

- *Media*. The media is to a health promotion professional as medicine is to a doctor, or a drawing board is to an architect. Action can occur, but success is made more difficult without the use of mass and/or limited-reach media. This includes traditional media such as TV, radio and the press, as well as new and emerging media channels such as the Internet, email, pay TV and so on (Egger, Donovan & Spark 1993).
- *Product/equipment*. Drugs for immunisation (e.g. filariasis in developing countries) would fit into this category. It could also include the use of new equipment such as pedometers for feedback about movement levels. Technological development means that new products are continually being developed that could be included as part of your equipment. A video and digital camera are also useful for capturing images that could be used in other media presentations, and a good-quality tape recorder is of value for focus groups.
- *Clinical tools*. There is a wide range of standard tools that can assist clinical practice. Most of these are related to behaviour change and modifying thought processes. They include, but are not limited to, basic 'barefoot clinician' skills, such as weight management, basic counselling skills and measurement techniques.
- *Environmental diagnosis (ANGELO)*. The ANGELO model (see chapter 7) is a tool for environmental diagnosis that also assists in involving a community in an intervention and providing basic education to key stakeholders. The technique was developed to assist in obesity management but could also be used for other health issues.
- *Capacity building*. This is particularly useful when working in developing countries or communities where up-skilling of professionals is likely to be an aid. It can include structured workshops, social marketing, health promotion strategies and method, quit smoking, infectious disease control and so on. Although some modifications might be needed for different audiences, the basic principles and objectives remain constant.
- *Interactive group workshops*. These include semi-structured programs for target groups in weight control, quitting smoking, drug use, healthy cooking, physical activity and so on. Again, some modifications might be necessary for different audiences.
- *Focus group sessions*. Focus groups are used as a form of formative research and to provide ideas for creative development of later interventions in a health promotion program. These have a semi-structured format with options for changing in the direction required as a result of participant input.
- *Personal assessment/risk factor measurement tools*. At the basic level these might include such equipment as weight and body fat scales and a tape measure that can be used for personal assessment as well as measurement for evaluation purposes. At a more sophisticated level it

could involve the use of a standard measurement protocol, such as the STEPS program, developed for measuring baseline and follow-up health indices in Pacific Island countries by the WHO (Bonita et al. 2001).

- *Questionnaires and survey materials.* A range of standard health questionnaires is available for use with individuals and populations. At the individual level, the use of diet diaries and dietary recall also provides an indication of food and nutrient intake in individuals and populations. Pedometers can be used in small samples to determine basic movement levels and to provide information about required levels.
- *Presentation tools.* Use of PowerPoint presentations and mobile projectors is vital for a range of the tasks required in health promotion, including communicating with the general public as well as health professionals. Small mobile computers and projectors now make this feasible.

Competencies required of the health promotion professional

The following table lists the main competencies seen as essential or desirable for health promotion professionals in Australia. It has been adapted from a review of competencies initially completed in 1994 and updated in 2003 (Shilton et al. 2003). Competencies have been listed under the headings provided in the SOPIE model discussed in chapter 9.

Situational analysis

Competencies include being able to:

1. identify behavioural, environmental and organisational factors that promote or compromise health
2. assist and involve communities in identifying needs and setting priorities for health promotion
3. identify and source data on health needs
4. critically analyse relevant literature.

Objective setting

Competencies include being able to:

1. formulate appropriate and measurable objectives
2. develop logical, sequenced and sustainable programs based on theory and evidence
3. communicate verbally and listen reflectively
4. debate health-related issues using evidence-based arguments

5. consider and apply theory to health promotion planning, implementation and research.

Planning

Competencies include being able to:

1. establish appropriate partnerships and facilitate collaborative action
2. involve community members and stakeholders in program planning and action
3. apply a range of approaches to health education
4. coordinate production of appropriate program support materials
5. liaise and collaborate with other professionals and organisations
6. use technology-based systems and resources such as the Internet.

Implementation

Competencies include being able to:

1. assist, support and build capacity in service providers and clinical workers
2. apply interpersonal skills (negotiation, teamwork, motivation, conflict resolution, decision making and problem solving)
3. apply mass media, group, healthy policy and structural/environmental strategies
4. write and apply interviewee skills for media
5. be able to articulate health promotion jargon into salient language
6. devolve programs to the community
7. work as part of a team.

Evaluation

Competencies include being able to:

1. identify appropriate evaluation designs
2. interpret and communicate evaluation findings
3. monitor programs and adjust objectives.

A final look: health promotion— the human factor

As with all vocations, certain skills, tools and competencies are seen as essential for the profession of health promotion. Although no single health promotion practitioner could be expected to be expert in all the skills and competencies discussed here, the wider the range available in any practitioner's repertoire, the greater the potential utility of that individual. Together with the strategies and methods discussed in this book, the skills, tools, and competencies discussed in this chapter help to define the requirements of a successful modern health promotion practitioner. They also provide a blueprint for modern health promotion. However, no program should ever underestimate the power of the human factor, or the person making it happen. To be fully successful, as well as happy in their chosen vocation, the true health promotion practitioner requires not just personal and process skills but also a more than adequate supply of 'fire in the belly'—a belief and commitment to the value of health promotion in contributing to improvements in human health—as well as improvements in the less specific, but equally important, area of quality of life.

References

Bonita, R., de Courten, M., Dwyer, T., Jamrozik, K., & Winkelmann, R., 2001, *Surveillance of Risk Factors for Noncommunicable Diseases: The WHO STEPwise Approach*, Summary, World Health Organization, Geneva.

Doll, R., Peto, R., Boreham, J., & Sutherland, I., 2004, 'Mortality in relation to smoking: 50 years' observations on male British doctors', *Brit Med J* 328:1519–30.

Egger, G., 2004, 'Health promotion consultant's instructional manual', unpublished WHO report.

Egger, G., Donovan, R. J., & Spark, R., 1993, *Health and the Media: Principles and Practice for Health Promotion*, McGraw-Hill, Sydney.

Shilton, T., Howat, P., James, R., & Lower, T., 2003, 'Review of competencies for Australian health promotion', *IUHPE—Promotion and Education* 10(4):162–70.

Index